Schering Foundation Workshop 5
Sex Steroids and the Cardiovascular System

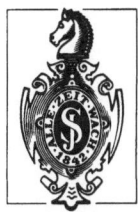

Schering Foundation Workshop

Editors: Günter Stock
Ursula-F. Habenicht

Schering Foundation Workshop 5

Sex Steroids and the Cardiovascular System

P. Ramwell, G. Rubanyi, E. Schillinger,
Editors

With 56 Figures

Springer-Verlag Berlin Heidelberg GmbH

ISBN 978-3-662-02766-0   ISBN 978-3-662-02764-6 (eBook)
DOI 10.1007/978-3-662-02764-6

© Springer-Verlag Berlin Heidelberg 1992
Originally published by Springer-Verlag Berlin Heidelberg New York in 1992
Softcover reprint of the hardcover 1st edition 1992
The use of general descriptive names, registered names, trademarks, etc. in this publication does not imply, even in the absence of a specific statement, that such names are exempt from the relevant protective laws and regulations and therefore free for general use.

Product liability: The publishers cannot guarantee the accuracy of any information about dosage and application contained in this book. In every individual case the user must check such information by consulting the relevant literature.

Typesetting: Data conversion by Springer-Verlag

21/3130-5 4 3 2 1 0 - Printed on acid-free paper

Preface

Evidence accumulated over the past decade show that gonadal steroid hormones participate in an important way in the physiological and pathophysiological regulation of the cardiovascular system. The hormonal profile appears to put males at a disadvantage biologically in terms of cardiovascular diseases. The incidence of hypertension is higher in men than in pre-monopausal women indicating an influence of gender on the hypertensive disease process. Males and females have equivalent cholesterol levels until puberty but males suffer an exponential increase in heart disease in their forties, while the female rise does not start until a decade later, after menopause. Animal and human studies provided ample evidence, that estrogens lower the levels of low density lipoproteins and keep high density lipoproteins elevated. These changes may be advantageous in the prevention of heart diesease. Coronary artery atherosclerosis has been shown to be more pronounced in ovarectomized female monkeys as in intact females. Androgen, conversely, lowers the high density lipoproteins and elevates low density lipoproteins. Regarding blood pressure, it is well established that hypertension is more severe or develops more rapidly in male than female rats in several genetic forms of hypertension, and that gonadal steroid hormones are probably playing an important role in explaining this observation. Risk factors of human hypertension and coronary heart diesease include menopause and ovarectomy.

Despite these convincing evidences from epidemiological and animal studies, there are presently few data to link menopause to the increased rate of hypertension or coronary heart disease. For example, studies on cellular mechanisms of atherosclerosis have been conducted predominantly in male animals. The mechanisms by which steroids may influence the proliferation of smooth muscle cells and plaque formation is unclear. Although endothelial injury, activation and consequent dysfunction is an important feature in both hypertension and atherogenesis, data are not available on gender differences in vascular wall response to injury, endothelial integrity or the proliferative response.

The Schering Foundation Workshop on "Sex Steroids and the Cardiovascular System", which took place in Berlin on February 5–7, 1992, was organized to discuss the present knowledge and future research directions in this important, but still poorly understood field. Leading basic scientists, epidemiologists and clinicians reviewed and discussed three main themes: Firstly, sexual dimorphism and the role of sex steroids (estrogen, progesterone and testosterone) in the control of the cardiovascular system and physiological (e.g. pregnancy) and pathological (e.g. hypertension) conditions; secondly, sex steroids and vascular wall biology and pathology, and thirdly, oral contraceptive steroids and hemostasis.

This book contains the proceedings of the workshop. The excellent chapters by the leading experts give an overview of the methodologies (from transgenic techniques to classical physiology methods) and the multidisciplinary approaches utilized to analyze some of the scientific questions.

In addition to the comprehensive summary of the present state of the art in these three areas, this book also points out basic questions where future research is needed. The organizers of the workshop and editors of this volume consider the latter as one of the major achievements of the meeting and hope that this book will stimulate scientists and clinicians alike to continue or initiate research in these and related areas.

Peter Ramwell
Gabor M. Rubanyi
Ekkehard Schillinger

Contents

List of Contributors

Abi-Younes, Sylvie
Department of Physiology and Biophysics, Georgetown University
Medical Center, 3800 Reservoir Road NW, Washington DC 20007,
USA

Adams, Michael R.
Comparative Medicine Clinical Research Center, Bowman Gray
School of Medicine of Wake Forest University, Medical Center Blvd.,
Winston-Salem, NC 27157

Bachmann, Jürgen
German Institute for High Blood Pressure Research, Im Neuenheimer
Feld 366, 6900 Heidelberg, FRG

Baldus, Berthold
Research Center of Schering AG, Müllerstr., 1000 Berlin 65, FRG

Chwalisz, Krzystof
Research Center of Schering AG, Müllerstr., 1000 Berlin 65, FRG

Clarkson, Thomas B.
Comparative Medicine Clinical Research Center, Bowman Gray
School of Medicine of Wake Forest University, Medical Center Blvd.,
Winston-Salem, NC 27157

Crofton, Joan T.
Department of Physiology and Biophysics, University of Tennessee, 894 Union Avenue, Memphis, TN 38163, USA

Farhat, Michel
Department of Physiology and Biophysics, Georgetown University Medical Center, 3800 Reservoir Road NW, Washington DC 20007, USA

Foegh, Marie L.
Department of Surgery, Georgetown University Medical Center, 3800 Reservoir Road NW, Washington DC 20007, USA

Fritzemeier, Karl-Heinrich
Research Center of Schering AG, Müllerstr., 1000 Berlin 65, FRG

Ganten, Detlef
Max Delbrück Center for Molecular Medicine (MDC), Robert-Rössle-Str. 10, 1115 Berlin Buch, FRG

Ganten, Ursula
Max Delbrück Center for Molecular Medicine (MDC), Robert-Rössle-Str. 10, 1115 Berlin Buch, FRG

Gevers Leuven, Jan A.
IVVO-TNO, Gaubius Laboratory, P.O. Box 430, 2300 AK Leiden, The Netherlands

Graf, Hermann
Institute of Pharmacology, Schering AG, Muellerstrasse 170-178, 1000 Berlin 65, FRG

Helmerhorst, Frans M.
University Hospital, 2300 AK Leiden, The Netherlands

Kluft, Cees
IVVO-TNO, Gaubius Laboratory, P.O. Box 430, 2300 AK Leiden, The Netherlands

Mammen, Eberhard F.
Departments of Obstetrics and Gynecology, Pathology and Physiology, Wayne State University School of Medicine, 275 East Hancock Avenue, Detroit, MI 48201, USA

Morton, Mark J.
Division of Cardiology, L464, Department of Medicine, Oregon Health Sciences University, 3181 SW Sam Jackson Park Road, Portland, OR 97201, USA

Parczyk, Karsten
Research Center of Schering AG, Müllerstr., 1000 Berlin 65, FRG

Ramey, Estelle
Department of Physiology and Biophysics, Georgetown University Medical Center, 3800 Reservoir Road NW, Washington D.C. 20007, USA

Ramwell, Peter W.
Department of Physiology and Biophysics, Georgetown University Medical Center, 3800 Reservoir Road NW, Washington DC 20007, USA

Share, Leonard
Department of Physiology and Biophysics, University of Tennessee, 894 Union Avenue, Memphis, TN 38163, USA

Stampfer, Meir J.
Channing Laboratory, Department of Medicine, Harvard Medical School, Brigham and Women's Hospital, 180 Longwood Avenue, Boston, MA 02115, USA

Stock, Günter
Schering AG, Müllerstr., 1000 Berlin 65, FRG

Süßmilch, Andreas
Research Center of Schering AG, Müllerstr., 1000 Berlin 65, FRG

Vargas, Roberto
Department of Physiology and Biophysics, Georgetown University Medical Center, 3800 Reservoir Road NW, Washington DC 20007, USA

Wagner, Janice D.
Comparative Medicine Clinical Research Center, Bowman Gray School of Medicine of Wake Forest University, Medical Center Blvd., Winston-Salem, NC 27157

Wolfe, Raymond M.
Department of Physiology and Biophysics, Georgetown University Medical Center, 3800 Reservoir Road NW, Washington DC 20007, USA

Zierz, Rupprecht
Research Center of Schering AG, Müllerstr., 1000 Berlin 65, FRG

1 Cardiovascular Sexual Dimorphism

Peter W. Ramwell and Estelle Ramey

1.1 Introduction

The assigned topic "cardiovascular sexual dimorphism" is difficult to review owing to the paucity of human data available. For example, virtually nothing is known of the differences in hemodynamics between young men and women. There is, in fact, an urgent need to improve understanding of how sex affects the prevention, diagnosis, and treatment of cardiovascular, cardiopulmonary, and thrombotic disease. The situation in women is complicated not only because of the menstrual cycle, pregnancy, and menopause but also because of additional factors not present with men such as the use of oral contraceptives and hormone replacement therapy. Another important cardiovascular factor in both sexes stems from sexual conditioning of behavior particularly aggression, which in its most extreme form is expressed by men in the U.S. being responsible for 95% of the murders of women. The issues of womens' health, especially in the cardiovascular field, are now being addressed seriously in the U.S. with the appointment of Dr. Bernadine Healy as Head of the NIH.

1.2 Sexual Dimorphic Distribution of Steroid Receptors

Jost, between 1947 and 1952, formulated the hypothesis relating genetic or chromosomal sex to gonadal sex, which leads to the sexual phenotype. Androgen is the major determinant of extragenital sexual dimorphism in that it promotes male phenotypic development. Although ovarian estrogen has a lesser role, it does have a major differentiating effect on the reproductive tract, fat distribution, and pelvic bones and thus give rise to the female phenotype. If androgen has the major differentiating effect, then one may anticipate the more widespread presence of androgen receptors in extragenital male tissue than estrogen receptors. However, little work has been done on the distribution of human sex steroid receptors (Campisi et al. 1987) other than on breast and prostate biopsies. What has been done is interesting and provocative. For example, there is a sexual dimorphism in androgen receptors in the human thyroid wherein only men and not women express these receptors (Sheridan et al. 1984). The significance of this observation is still obscure. More recently an interesting deficiency in the androgen receptor gene which is normally expressed by spinal and bulbar motoneurones has been observed in a rat model of the muscular dystrophy characteristic of Kennedy's disease (La Spada et al. 1991). In patients it appears that these motoneurones may lack the X-linked androgen receptor without any evidence of a decrease in the androgen receptor expression associated with testicular feminization syndrome. Some cases of this latter syndrome are recently described to be linked to a complete absence of the androgen receptor gene in the cells studied. This lack of androgen receptor genes in these very different diseases suggest the existence of different androgen receptors.

1.3 Testosterone and Cardiovascular Disease

The putative role of testosterone, in the higher morbidity and mortality expressed by the male was first discussed by Hamilton 1948. In a most remarkable review he postulated that testosterone was a risk factor in males throughout the mammalian animal kingdom. As a result we tested the effect of sex, testosterone and estradiol treatment in a number of animal models. We showed that male sex and testosterone treatment increased mortality in a murine "sudden death" model (Uzanova et al. 1977). In a rodent occlusive arterial thrombosis model we found maleness to be significantly deleterious and testosterone to dramatically increase thrombosis in both sexes. It may be important to note that subcutaneously administered estradiol significantly reduced thrombosis (Uzanova et al. 1976; Leovey et al. 1980). In this model, thrombosis develops in a plastic loop inserted into the abdominal aorta. The data indicate that estradiol may have a beneficial antithrombotic effect on the blood elements but not necessarily on the vascular wall. However, at present there is no conclusive evidence that male sex per se in man is a risk factor in the pathogenesis of arterial thrombogenesis although coronary plaque formation and consequently plaque rupture are greater in men than postmenopausal women. Blood coagulability and estrogen will be discussed elsewhere in this symposium.

The major cause of death in both sexes is vascular disease. Within the cardiovascular category, there are large sex differences with respect to morbidity and the age at onset of coronary disease. Hypertension is a primary risk factor. For example, prior to menopause, women have lower blood pressure than men but become more hypertensive after menopause. There are many likely reasons for the lower blood pressure in young women. In contrast to men, young women are remarkably free of coronary heart disease, until menopause. One may speculate that this is related to the marked sex difference in lipid metabolism in the child-bearing years, during which the female metabolism is directed to providing the fetus with glucose from fatty acids. To what extent this relates to sex differences in hemodynamics is not known. In a rodent model we found that pressor responses to norepinephrine were exaggerated by testosterone and the male sex (Baker et al. 1978, Baker et al. 1980).

The special consideration of women with respect to coronary heart disease was not extensively reviewed until 1988 when it was done by (Murdaugh et al 1988). They conclude that significant differences do indeed exist in the clinical manifestations of coronary heart disease in the two sexes with respect to the specificity and sensitivity of noninvasive tests, differences in the age at which medical care is sought, in morbidity and mortality, differences in pharmacotherapy, and also differences in outcome of percutaneous transluminal angioplasty and coronary artery bypass graft procedures. In addition there are serious difficulties due to exclusion or under-representation of women in both small and large clinical trials, which is a problem currently addressed by NIH guidelines.

1.4 Sexual Dimorphism of the Immune System

Of particular interest to us is whether there are sex differences in accelerated coronary artery atherosclerosis in organ transplants and following endothelial damage during angioplasty. This issue has been addressed by Marie Foegh (this volume). However, in terms of organ rejection it is thought that women cardiac recipients reject organs more frequently and earlier than male patients (Esmore et al. 1991). This may also relate to the fact that there is more graft versus host disease in male bone marrow recipients of female bone marrow. This argues that in both cases the immune system is more expressed in women than in men. The higher incidence of autoimmune disease such as lupus erythematosus in women also speak to the more vigorous nature of the female immune response (Denman 1991). Interestingly the immune response to the allograft is attenuated in renal transplant patients by pregnancy, so much so that the dose of the immunosupressant drugs can be reduced up to the time of delivery, at which time they must immediately be administered at the full dose. It would be of interest to determine the effect of hormone replacement therapy in non pregnant patients both on the allograft as well as on attendant autoimmune disease. Pregnancy is well known to be associated with spontaneous remission of rheumatoid arthritis which has an incidence of 4:1 in women and men.

There is a prominent sex difference in phagocytosis by monocytes, which in women is increased further by both estrogen and by pregnancy. Monocyte-macrophages are thought to have a significant role in the development of atherosclerosis and the foam cell. It is possible that the sexual dimorphism in atherosclerosis may relate to the sexual dimorphism observed in these cells. This sexual dimorphism is readily demonstrated in elicited rat peritoneal macrophages where differences in arachidonate cyclooxygenase can be measured (Du et al. 1984). There is also a sexual dimorphism in cyclooxygenase products in human polymorphonucleocytes (Mallery et al. 1986).

In addition to hemodynamics, the immune system, and lipid metabolism there are major sex differences in hormonal patterns as, for example, in the release of growth hormone, ACTH, cortisol and catecholamines which may relate to myocardial infarction which peaks in men in the morning hours but not in women. An increased pattern of occurrence of stroke in the morning hours has also been described but a circadian difference between men and women has not been demonstrated.

1.5 Sexual Dimorphism of the Neuro-Endocrine System

Of particular interest are the neuromorphological differences currently being identified using scanners. The larger corpus callosum in women and the presence of the sexually dimorphic nucleus in men are provocative findings. Although work in animals is well advanced, the sexual differentiation of specific brain function in men and women and its relation to cardiovascular disease is only beginning to be addressed. One of the most important factors may be the sex differences in growth hormone release which regulates the phenotype of the liver, which is reflected in sex differences in enzymatic activity and protein synthesis. The episodic nature of the growth hormone secretory pattern is directly linked to sex steroid masculinization of the neonatal brain. The sexually differentiated secretory pattern accounts at least in part for the sex differences in body growth as well as liver function. Clinically, estrogens antagonize several effects of growth hormone. Whether this sexual differentiation leads to sex differences in vascular growth factors after injury is interesting. Our efforts to show sex differences in myointimal proliferation have not been successful. It is some of these consideration which has led us to explore somatostatin, another hypothalamic hormone, as an inhibitor of growth hormone release and as a potential inhibitor of vascular growth factors. Our data show that a stable octapeptide analog of somatostatin does indeed inhibit myointimal proliferation in a wide range of different animal models and also on coronary artery segments in vitro. Phase II-III clinical studies are in progress for inhibition of restenosis after coronary artery angioplasty.

1.6 Inheritance and Sexual Dimorphism

It may be of special significance that inheritance of mitochondrial DNA appears to be an exclusive maternal mode of inheritance (Gyllensten et al. 1991). This speaks to the work by Capasso and his colleagues, who find larger mitochondria and more active oxidative phosphorylation in myocardial tissue (Capasso et al. 1983) and in cytochrome in murine renal tissue from males than from females. This is an interesting point in that it recalls Hamilton's conclusion that males generally have higher body temperatures and Q_{O2} than females. Men posses thyroid androgen receptors and women do not.

Another anabolic hormone which interacts synergistically with other hormones and growth factors to promote growth and proliferation in insulin. There is an important sex difference in insulin secretion in response to a glucose load in men and women. This may be yet another factor which with cholesterol and all the others incrementally favor the women's cardiovascular system.

1.7 Conclusion

In conclusion, it is clear that there is need to develop a data base on the relevant factors relating to sexual dimorphism of the cardiovascular system. The situation is difficult due to the observation made in women without allowing for the variables in women's lives as already described. For example, the internal mammary artery is of great utility in bypass surgery in both sexes. Is there a difference in functionality between vessels taken from men and from women who breastfed their children? Further, will estrogen treatment prior to and following surgery improve graft function in postmenopausal women? Clearly, such questions are relevant to improving women's health in the future. What we need for men is a nonfeminizing estrogen.

References

Baker PJ, Ramey ER, Ramwell PW (1978) Androgen-mediated sex differences of cardiovascular responses in rats. Am. J. Physiol. 235:242-246

Baker PJ, Ramey ER, Ramwell PW (1980) Sex differences in vascular responses to arachidonic acid. In: Prostaglandins in cardiovascular and renal function. , Scriabine A, Lefer A, and Kuehl FA (eds.). Spectrum Publications, New York, pp. 363

Campisi D, Bivona A, Paterna S, Valenza M, Albiero R (1987) Oestrogen binding in fresh human aortic tissue. Int J Tiss Reac IX:5,393-398

Capasso JM, Remily RM, Smith RH, Sonnenblick EH (1983) Sex differences in myocardial contractility in the rat. Basic Res Cardiol. 78:156-171

Denman AM (1991) Sex hormones, autoimmune diseases, and immune responses. BMJ 303:2-3

Du JT, Vennos E, Ramey E, Ramwell PW (1984) Sex differences in arachidonate cyclo-oxygenase products in elicited rat peritoneal macrophages. Biochemica et Biophysica Acta 794:256-260

Esmore D, Keogh A, Spratt P, Jones B, Chang V (1991) Heart Transplantation in females. J Heart Lung Transpl 10:335-341

Gyllensten U, Wharton D, Josefsson A, Wilson AC (1991) Paternal inheritance of mitochondral DNA in mice. Nature 352:255-257

Hamilton JB (1948) The role of testicular secretion as indicated by the effects of castration in man and by studies of pathological conditions and the short lifespan associated with maleness. Recent Prog Horm Res 3:247

La Spada, AR, Wilson EM, Lubahn DB, Harding AE, Fischbeck KH (1991) Androgen receptor gene mutation in x-linked spinal and bulbar muscular atrophy. Nature 352:77-79

Leovey EMK, Ramey ER, Maddox Y, Ramwell PW (1980) Sex and gonadal steroid effects on arachidonate uptake into rat platelets. Adv Prostaglandin Thromb Res 8:1277

Mallery SR, Zeligs BJ, Ramwell PW, Bellanti JA (1986) Gender-related variations and interaction of human neutrophil cyclooxygenase and oxidative burst metabolites. J Leukocyte Biol 40:133-146

Murdaugh CL, O'Rourke RA (1988) Coronary heart disease in women: Special considerations. Curr Probl Cardiol 13:73-156

Sheridan PJ, McGill HC Jr, Lissitzky JC, Martin PM (1984) The primate thyroid gland contains receptors for androgens. Endocrinology 115:2154-2159

Uzanova A, Ramey E, Ramwell PW (1976) Effect of testosterone, sex and age on experimentally induced arterial thrombosis. Nature 261:712

Uzanova A, Ramey E, Ramwell PW (1977) Arachidonate-induced thrombosis in mice: Effects of gender or testosterone or estradiol administration. Prostaglandins 13:955

2 Sexual Dimorphism of Cardiovascular Function: The Role of Androgens

Jürgen Bachmann, Ursula Ganten, Günter Stock, and Detlev Ganten

2.1 Introduction

Large-scale epidemiological studies have shown that the level of blood pressure is lower in women before menopause than in men (HDFP Cooperative Group 1977; Dawber 1980; Eiff et al. 1986; Cirillo and Trevisan 1992). Likewise, the prevalence of hypertension is considerably lower in premenopausal women than in men. In women after menopause, however, blood pressure levels and the prevalence of hypertension exceed the levels in men (Cirillo and Trevisan 1992). The generally held belief for this gender discrepancy is that ovarian hormones provide protection against cardiovascular disease. However, there is increasing evidence that testosterone and its metabolite dihydrotestosterone have an important effect on blood pressure and cardiovascular control mechanisms. Animal studies have shown that blood pressure is higher in genetically hypertensive male rats of different strains (Cambotti et al. 1984; Ganten et al. 1989; Ashton and Balment 1991) and in genetically hypertensive mice (Schlager and Weibust 1967; Schlager 1968), as well as in deoxycorticosterone (DOC)-salt hypertensive rats (Share et al. 1988), in which hypertension is induced by unilateral nephrectomy followed by subcutaneous administration of the mineralocorticoid DOC and 1% NaCl in the drinking water, a form of hypertension which requires the presence of vasopressin (Crofton et al. 1979). Blood pressure and related parameters like heart rate and relative changes in response to stress or sodium loading displayed considerable sexual dimorphism in F_1 (Ely and Turner 1990) and F_2 generations (Lindpaintner et al. 1990) of crosses between spontaneously hypertensive rats (SHR) or spontaneously hypertensive stroke-prone rats (SHRSP) and their respective control strains. In normotensive rats, however, blood pressure is not significantly different between males and females (Ganten et al. 1989; Ashton and Balment 1991). Thus the sexual dimorphism with respect to blood pressure in hypertensive rats provides an excellent model for further studies on the cellular and genetic basis of hypertension (Ganten et al. 1989; Wagner et al. 1990). Although the underlying mechanisms for the sex-related differences in blood pressure are not completely understood, there is much evidence for an important role of testosterone and estrogens for the development of this gender discrepancy. In this report, the effects of androgens on the cardiovascular system at different levels of its organization are reviewed. We will mainly analyze the influence of testosterone on components of the renin-angiotensin system in different tissues, since accumulating evidence suggests a central role of this system in the regulation of cardiovascular function and disease.

2.2 Metabolism and Receptor Binding of Testosterone in Target Cells

The metabolism of testosterone is shown in Fig. 1. Testosterone, the principal circulating androgen in the male, is secreted into the blood by testicular Leydig cells under luteinizing hormone (LH) stimulation. In the blood, it is either bound to albumin or to the sex hormone binding globulin (SHBG), a hepatic secreted protein that binds primarily testosterone and other 17β-hydroxylated steroids, including estradiol (Dunn et al. 1981), or to albumin. Testosterone enters the cell mainly by diffusion. In the cell, the steroid can react in the following ways (Bardin and Catteral 1981):

1. Without being metabolized, it binds directly to the androgen receptor in the nucleus, and this steroid receptor complex reacts with nuclear acceptor sites in chromatin for initiation of the steroid-specific responses.
2. Testosterone is metabolized by 5α-reductase to 5α-dihydrotestosterone which then binds to the androgen receptor. The steroid receptor complex then reacts with nuclear acceptor sites in the nucleus; 5α-dihydrotestosterone, which cannot be aromatized to estrogen, exhibits a higher affinity to the androgen receptor than testosterone and is two to three times more potent than testosterone (Toscano 1986).
3. Testosterone is aromatized to estradiol which binds to the estrogen receptor. The steroid-receptor complex is bound to the nucleus for initiation of estrogen-specific responses.
4. Testosterone is metabolized to 5β-metabolites which bind to the β-steroid receptor and the steroid-receptor complex presumably acts in the nucleus.
5. Testosterone or its metabolites act in the nucleus or cytoplasm by receptor-independent mechanisms. One example is the action of the steroid on the pentose phosphate cycle of the prostate which is mediated by cyclic AMP.

In the nucleus, the steroid-receptor complex binds to specific acceptor sites located in the 5'region of specific DNA sequences to initiate transcription (Clark et al. 1985). Acceptor sites distant to the structural gene which is activated have been described (Theveny et al. 1987) and involve the formation of DNA loops which allow binding of specific transcription factors. The control of gene expression by steroid hormones may either be exerted by direct interaction with a structural gene or by activation of an integrator gene which then synthesizes an activator molecule, for example, RNA or protein, that induces gene expression of one or several structural genes. Moreover, posttranscrip-

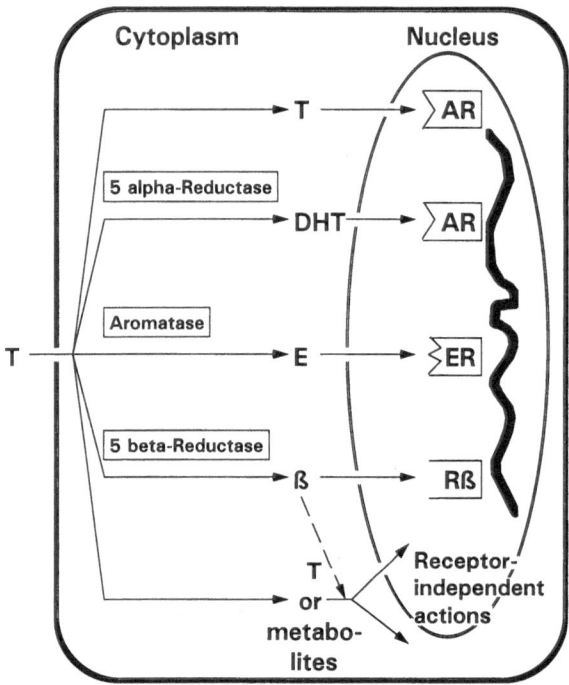

Fig. 1. Metabolism and receptor binding of testosterone in target cells. Testosterone (*T*) leaves the blood and enters the target cell by diffusion. In the cytoplasm, the steroid can react in the following ways: (a) It passes the cytoplasm and binds to the androgen receptor (*AR*) in the nucleus. (b) T is metabolized by the enzyme 5α-reductase to 5α-dihydrotestosterone (*DHT*) which enters the nucleus and binds to AR. (c) T is aromatized to estradiol (*E*) which binds to the estrogen receptor (*ER*). (d) T is metabolized to 5β metabolites which bind to the β steroid receptor (*Rβ*). (e) T or one of its metabolites act in the nucleus or cytoplasm by receptor-independent mechanisms. (a-e) After binding of T or its metabolites to steroid receptors, the steroid receptor complex reacts with nuclear acceptor sites to initiate transcription of specific genes

tional mechanisms concerning the control of cell function by steroid hormones have been described. These mechanisms include stabilization of mRNA or modulation of translation (McKnight and Palmiter 1979; Brock and Shapiro 1983; Fulton and Birnie 1985; Berger et al. 1986).

2.3 Effects of Testosterone on Blood Pressure
in Genetically Hypertensive Rats

Phoenix et al. (1959) showed that androgens had direct effects on the brain. They suggested that during early development androgens act to organize neural pathways responsible for male behaviours, while in adults, androgens act on differentiated pathways to activate previously organized behaviors. It was shown that in rodents, the gonadal hormone pattern during the neonatal period influences sexual brain differentiation (McEwen 1981; Wilson et al. 1981; Mooradian et al. 1987). To test for the hypothesis that the neonatal gonadal hormonal environment establishes the sexually dimorphic pattern of hypertension development in SHR, Cambotti et al. (1984) castrated male spontaneously hypertensive rats (SHR) on the day of birth and administered testosterone to 2-day-old female SHR and followed up their blood pressure development. They found that orchidectomy lowered blood pressure to the level of control female SHR and testosterone treatment of females increased blood pressure to the level of control males. Testosterone implants in adult rats increased blood pressure of control male and neonatally androgenized female SHR, whereas in control females and neonatally castrated males, blood pressure remained constant during testosterone treatment in adulthood. The authors concluded that the presence or absence of testosterone in the neonatal period served as a sufficient condition for the development of the male or female hypertensive pattern, respectively, and determined the response threshold to postpubertal testosterone. Testosterone may therefore directly alter the organization of brain areas in which neuropeptides with cardiovascular effects are produced, for example, in the hypothalamus and the caudal medulla. The important question of whether the effects of testosterone on the organization of brain areas involved in cardiovascular regulation are dependent on aromatization or 5α-reduction of testosterone cannot be decided yet. Aromatization of testosterone to estradiol varies from region to region. The enzymatic activity is absent from the pituitary and cerebral cortex but present in the hippocampus, amygdala, and preoptic area (McEwen 1980). The activity of 5α-reductase, however, is distributed throughout the central nervous system and, thus, does not appear to be a limiting factor in androgen occupancy of receptors (McEwen 1980). Interestingly, 5α-reductase activity is higher perinatally than in the adult, suggesting an important role for dihydrotestosterone in neuronal organization (Rees and Michael 1984; Bonsall et al. 1985; Michael et al. 1986). Androgen receptors in brain tissues have similar physicochemical properties to those of the prostate, recognizing both testosterone and dihydrotestosterone (Christensen and Gorski 1978). In primates and rodents, the majority of androgen receptors was found in the pituitary, hypothalamus, preoptic area, septum, and amygdala, with the lowest concentration being in the cerebellum (McEwen 1980; Tobet et al. 1985). Thus, androgen receptors are present in regions which play an important role in the regulation of cardiovascular function (Mangiapane et al. 1989).

The results of Cambotti et al. (1984) were confirmed by Ganten et al. (1989) who found that surgical castration of neonatal male SHR reduced blood pressure to the female level (Fig. 2a). Moreover, SHR were treated with the androgen receptor antagonists flutamide, which causes a feedback elevation of plasma testosterone (Neri and Kassem 1984) or cyproterone acetate (CPA), an androgen receptor antagonist which does not lead to an increase of circulating testosterone levels (Neumann and Kramer 1966; Neumann and Hasan 1980), for a period of 10 days following parturition. This treatment, which was shown to inhibit male brain maturation and subsequently male behavior in rats (Neumann and Steinbeck 1972), also markedly reduced hypertension development in male SHR (Fig. 2a). Surgical castration of male SHR at 4 (Iams and Wexler 1979) or male SHRSP at 9 weeks of age (Ganten et al. 1989), and the blockade of androgen receptors in SHRSP with flutamide from 8 to 17 weeks of age, i.e., during the developmental phase of hypertension in prepuberty and puberty, efficiently reduced blood pressure (Fig. 2b) (Ganten et al. 1989). However, surgical

Fig. 2a-c. Effects of castration and antiandrogen treatment on blood pressure of SHR and SHRSP of different age. **a** Reduction of blood pressure in 13-weeks-old male SHR castrated neonatally (*Orchid.*) or treated with cyproterone acetate (*CPA*) or flutamide (*Flut.*) for 10 days following parturition. **b** Effect of flutamide treatment or orchidectomy on blood pressure of young male SHRSP. Rats were either treated with flutamide for 2 months starting at 8 weeks of age or orchidectomized at 9 weeks. Blood pressure was measured weekly until 20 weeks of age. The results of a recording at 17 weeks of age are shown here. **c** Surgical or chemical castration in 25-week-old male SHR. Blood pressure was not significantly different among the groups

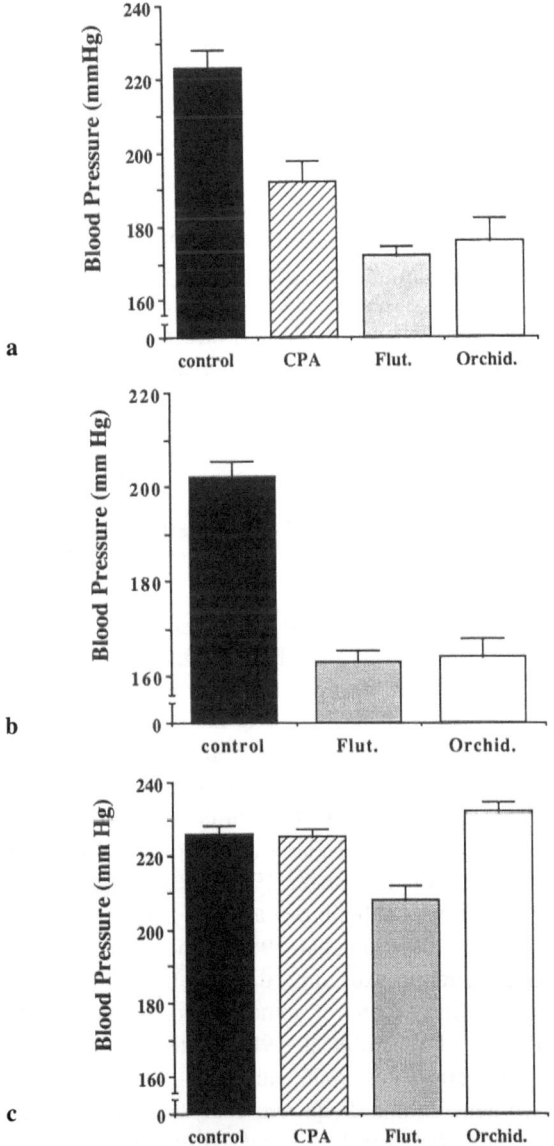

castration of male SHR postpubertally either at 12 (Cambotti et al. 1984) or 25 weeks (Ganten et al. 1989) or androgen receptor blockade at 25 weeks (Ganten et al. 1989) did not influence blood pressure (Fig. 2c). There are two possible explanations for these observations. On the one hand, the critical period for organizational effects of androgens on hypothalamic areas and the vascular system for future sex differences in hypertensive patterns may extend beyond the neonatal stage into prepuberty. This is unlikely since it was shown (Rhees et al. 1990) that the sensitive period during which exogenous androgen administration determines male brain differentiation of sensitive nuclei is limited to 5 days following parturition. On the other hand, testosterone may affect blood pressure development in genetically hypertensive male rats via direct hormone receptor-mediated mechanisms. This possibility is of particular interest in view of the fact that steroids directly act on gene expression (Fig. 1).

2.4 Regulation of Tissue Renin-Angiotensin Systems by Testosterone

Since the renin-angiotensin system (RAS) is centrally involved in the regulation of blood pressure and fluid homeostasis (Hackenthal et al. 1990), its components renin, angiotensinogen, angiotensin converting enzyme (ACE), and angiotensin II receptor are candidate genes for the development of hypertension. Besides its well-defined role as an endocrine system, evidence is increasing for local RAS in several tissues (Paul et al. 1992), including brain (Ganten et al. 1983; Ganten et al. 1984; Fuxe et al. 1988), adrenal gland (Urata et al. 1988; Oda et al. 1991), kidney (Dzau and Ingelfinger 1989), heart (Lindpaintner and Ganten 1991), vasculature (Schelling et al. 1991), and reproductive organs (Parmentier et al. 1983; Do et al. 1988; Daud et al. 1990).

Large amounts of renin, exceeding those in the kidney, have been found in the submaxillary gland of some mouse strains, e.g., DBA/2, Swiss or NMRI mice (Wilson et al. 1981). These "high-renin mice" carry two distinct renin genes (*Ren*-1 and *Ren*-2) and have therefore been termed two-gene strains. Sequence analysis of renin mRNA revealed 96% homology between *Ren*-1 and *Ren*-2 in the coding regions of these genes (Holm et al. 1984). *Ren*-2 is expressed, on the average, at 150-fold higher levels than *Ren*-1 in the submaxillary gland. In the mouse salivary gland, androgens are powerful stimulants of renin protein (Oliver and Gross 1967) and mRNA (Pratt et al. 1984), both in one-gene and in two-gene strains. Nuclear run-on assays have shown that the stimulation of renin mRNA by testosterone in the salivary gland is due to transcriptional regulation (Tronik and Rougeon 1988). Experiments performed in our laboratory showed that the stimulatory influence of androgens on renin is not limited to the salivary gland. Treatment of NMRI mice, which carry two renin genes, with dihydrotestosterone-stimulated renin mRNA in the submandibular gland, adrenal gland, brain, and heart (Metzger et al. 1988; Wagner et al. 1990). Interestingly, in the adrenal gland, renin mRNA increased already 2 h after testosterone administration, whereas in the brain, a significant stimulation of renin mRNA was found after 21 days of treatment. A possible explanation for these observations is that local renin-angiotensin systems respond in a tissue-specific manner to dihydrotestosterone administration and that different tissues participate in a differentiated way with respect to time, mechanism, and magnitude of renin stimulation. In the rat anterior pituitary gland, immunoreactive renin and angiotensin II were found within the same cells (Naruse et al. 1986). The intensity of renin immunoreactivity was higher in the male than in the female, and positive staining of renin was abolished by orchidectomy and restored by simultaneous administration of testosterone. These results provide evidence for the existence of a local pituitary RAS and for androgenic control of pituitary renin. In view of the strong experimental support for a renin-angiotensin system in the brain (Ganten et al. 1978; Slater et al. 1980; Okamura et al. 1981; Fishman et al. 1981), these results may reflect an increased local production of angiotensin II which has been shown to increase the release of vasopressin and ACTH (Malvin 1971; Mouw et al. 1971; Keil et al. 1975; Ramsay et al. 1978). Sexual differences in the activity of local RAS in these endocrine organs may modulate the production of hormones involved in blood pressure control. Such a mechanism could also contribute to the sexual dimorphism with respect to blood pressure. Other components of the RAS also show a tissue-specific stimulation by androgens. In the kidney, the mRNA of angiotensinogen is strongly increased by testosterone both in SHR and in WKY (Hellmann et al. 1988; Ellison et al. 1989). This observation is of particular interest in view of the local production of angiotensinogen in the proximal tubulus (Ingelfinger et al. 1990) and the sodium-retaining properties of angiotensin II (Cogan 1990). It has been suggested that local production of angiotensin II by a renal RAS (Gomez et al. 1988; Dzau and Ingelfinger 1989; Pratt et al. 1989) leads to increased sodium reabsorption via stimulation of the Na^+/H^+ antiport (Cogan 1990) which is localized in the proximal tubulus, too. The concept of a local renal RAS is supported by the observation that the concentration of angiotensin II is 100 times higher in the proximal tubulus than in the plasma (Seikaly et al. 1990). Thus the sexual dimorphism with respect to angiotensinogen production in the kidney may contribute to enhanced sodium absorption and to higher blood pressure in males. In the adrenal gland, an interaction of testosterone with angiotensin II receptors has been demonstrated. Testosterone was shown to increase the binding of angiotensin II and angiotensin III in bovine adrenal glomerulosa cells, and to stimulate basal and angiotensin-induced aldosterone production (Carroll and Goodfriend 1984).

2.5 Transgenic Animals: New Models to Study the Sexual Dimorphism with Regard to Blood Pressure

We investigated the question of whether the stimulatory influence of testosterone and dihydrotestosterone on the renin gene, which was found mainly in experiments with mice, is indeed relevant for blood pressure control. Since it is difficult to perform reliable hemodynamic analyses in mice, we addressed this question by introducing the entire murine *Ren*-2 gene including 5.3 and 9.5 kb of the 5' and 3' flanking sequence, respectively, into the genome of normotensive rats by microinjection. The founder animals carrying the transgene were severely hypertensive and transmitted both the transgene and the hypertensive phenotype to their progeny (Mullins et al. 1990). The transgenic rat line TGR(mREN2)27 developed fulminant hypertension. Surprisingly, active renin and angiotensin II in plasma are suppressed in TGR(mREN2)27 suggesting an important role of local tissue RAS for hypertension in these animals (Mullins et al. 1990; Ganten et al. 1991; Bader et al. 1992).

Moreover, TGR(mREN2)27 develop a marked sex difference with regard to the hypertensive phenotype, males exhibiting about 60 mm Hg higher blood pressure than females (Fig. 3a). In view of the

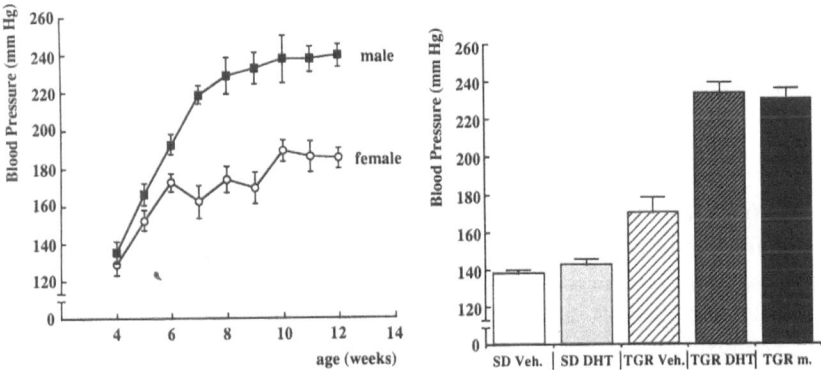

Fig. 3. *Left*, sexual dimorphism with regard to the development of hypertension in heterozygous TGR(mREN2)27. *Right*, effect of dihydrotestosterone (*DHT*) or vehicle (*Veh.*) treatment on blood pressure of young female TGR(mREN2)27 (*TGR*) and Sprague Dawley rats (*SD*). Treatment started at 5 weeks of age. The results of a recording at 11 weeks of age are shown. Male rats (*TGR m.*) were also vehicle treated

stimulatory effects of androgens on renin mRNA in mice, and since it was this mouse *Ren*-2 gene which was introduced into the genome of the transgenic rats TGR(mREN2)27 and produced fulminant hypertension, we examined whether androgens are important for this gender discrepancy. In a first set of experiments, we treated 5-week-old female TGR(mREN2)27 with dihydrotestosterone. The treated animals showed an accelerated development of hypertension, and their blood pressure reached the level of male TGR(mREN2)27. In contrast, dihydrotestosterone did not significantly change blood pressure of normotensive Sprague-Dawley rats (Fig. 3b). In adult female TGR(mREN2)27, however, dihydrotestosterone treatment did not modify blood pressure. Castration of 4-week-old male TGR(mREN2)27 significantly attenuated and reduced the development of hypertension. The experiments performed in TGR(mREN2)27 thus show that these transgenic rats provide a useful model system to investigate the role of local tissue RAS in the pathophysiology leading to the sexual dimorphism concerning blood pressure and hypertension. The importance of the renin-angiotensin system for the development of the sex difference in blood pressure is

further supported by the fact that transgenic mice carrying the rat angiotensinogen gene under control of its natural promotor also show a
marked sexual dimorphism with regard to blood pressure, with higher
blood pressure in males (Kimura et al. 1992).

2.6 Humoral Systems Involved in Blood Pressure Control: Modulation by Testosterone

The interaction of androgens with other humoral systems involved in
cardiovascular regulation at different levels of its organization have to
be considered as well. Testosterone modulates norepinephrine storage
and release in sympathetic fibers innervating vas deferens (Lara et al.
1985). In autoradiographic studies with [^{3}H]dihydrotestosterone, neural nuclear labeling has been found in brain areas, e.g., lower brain
stem, area postrema, basal hypothalamus and preoptic region (Stumpf
1990). These regions of the brain are involved in the control of blood
pressure and heart rate (Buggy and Fisher 1976; Diz and Jacobowitz
1984; Skoog and Mangiapane 1988; Mangiapane et al. 1989). Thus,
testosterone may directly modulate production of neuropeptides in the
anterior hypothalamus and the caudal medulla. Co-localization of
[^{3}H]dihydrotestosterone nuclear binding with monoamine and peptide
messengers has consistently been observed. Dihydrotestosterone and
catecholamine co-localization has been found in 50–80% of catecholamine neurons in the medulla oblongata, in the locus coeruleus, in the
region of the lemniscus lateralis, and in the nuclei arcuatus et periven-
tricularis hypothalami (Heritage et al. 1980).

It is well established that blood concentrations of steroid hormones
modulate vascular responses to oxytocin, vasopressin, norepinephrine
and epinephrine (Lloyd 1959; Altura 1975; St-Louis et al. 1986; Share
et al. 1988). These variations involve both release of vasoactive sub-
stances and receptor-mediated action. The gender discrepancy of vasopressin release in rats is abolished by gonadectomy and restored by
treatment of males with testosterone and females with ovarian hormones (Share et al. 1988). In rats, pressure responsiveness to vasopressin is higher in males than in cycling females in the diestrus, proestrus or metestrus phase of the estrus cycle, while it is identical in
males (Share et al. 1988) and in females in estrus. It remains to be

clarified why pressure responsiveness to vasopressin is higher in intact male rats, and why DOC-salt hypertension is attenuated by orchidectomy. It is also unexplained as yet why pressure responsiveness is greater in female rats in estrus, compared to other stages of the estrus cycle, while in DOC-salt treated rats, hypertension is exacerbated by ovariectomy but prevented by estradiol treatment.

Testosterone has been demonstrated to increase vascular reactivity to norepinephrine in spinal cats (Bhargava et al. 1967) and the perfused hindlimb of dogs (Greenberg et al. 1974). Similarly, treatment of orchidectomized rats with testosterone potentiated the vasopressor action of norepinephrine (Baker et al. 1978). In contrast, treatment with estradiol in castrated males produced no significant change in the response to norepinephrine. Moreover, gender has an important influence on vasorelaxing systems. Castration led to elevated levels of renal prostaglandin E_2 (Matsudaira et al. 1985), which acts as a vasodilator and may be a determinant of blood pressure (Needleman et al. 1974; Dunham 1976). It has been suggested that renal prostaglandin E_2 may be part of a gonad-mediated blood pressure regulation system. Baker et al. (1978) observed sex differences in the systemic depressor response to arachidonic acid in Sprague-Dawley rats and a reduction of this response by castration both in females and in males. Moreover, castrate males pretreated with testosterone 5 or 7 days previously gave a response to arachidonate infusion that was of the same order as that obtained with intact males, whereas administration of estradiol to orchidectomized rats did not cause any significant change in the depressor response to arachidonate. These results are interesting with regard to the fact that thromboembolic responses to arachidonate are evoked more readily in male than in female mice, a response which is exaggerated by exogenous androgens (Uzunova et al. 1976).

One reason for the sex differences concerning pressor responsiveness may be androgen-mediated alterations in the composition of the vascular wall. Mural fibrous proteins, elastin, and collagen, are significantly increased in androgen-treated animals (Wolinsky 1972). Conversely, Fischer (1972) observed that administration of estradiol to ovariectomized female rats reduced the accumulation of both collagen and elastin in the aorta. Further work by Fischer and Swain (1977) also showed that testosterone has an opposite, but less marked, effect on vascular connective tissue than estradiol. The aortas of castrated male rats that received estradiol exhibited significantly lower collagen, elastin, and collagen-to-elastin ratio and a higher percentage of elastin than the aortas of rats receiving testosterone. These results indicate that testosterone may cause a decrease in the distensibility of blood vessels by modulation of the connective tissue content and the ratio of collagen to elastin in the vessel wall. Moreover, it has been shown that testosterone has an anabolic effect on components of blood vessels, for example, vascular smooth muscle. This effect may potentiate the pressor response to norepinephrine and reduce the distensibility of male blood vessels. For example, Piper and Vane (1969) and Baker et al. (1978) observed that aortic strips of male rabbits were more responsive to vasoconstrictor agents than that of the females. More recently, Cunard et al. (1987) found that the vascular endothelium of male and female rats differed with respect to its relaxing potency. Male endothelium released significantly lower levels of vasodilator factors than the endothelium of females.

2.7 Testosterone and the Heart

Other investigators reported about the effects of testosterone on the heart. For example, work by Salt (1972) in the perfused rat heart showed that testosterone significantly inhibited both norepinephrine uptake and inactivation by cardiac tissue. Schaible et al. (1984) measured coronary flow, myocardial oxygen consumption and pump and muscle function in isolated working heart preparations taken from castrated animals and found an impairment of left ventricular filling and function (Schaible et al. 1984; Scheuer et al. 1987). These functional alterations were associated with depressed myofibrillar ATPase activity and a shift of the myosin isoenzyme pattern to the V_3 form. In male SHRSP rats, blood pressure decreased after gonadectomy and was accelerated by dihydrotestosterone substitution of gonadectomized rats (Lengsfeld et al. 1988). In addition, heart and body weight were significantly diminished in the gonadectomized animals. Dihydrotestosterone reversed this effect. Gonadectomy shifted the myosin isoenzyme pattern to the V_3 form while dihydrotestosterone replacement led to a myosin isoenzyme pattern in favor of the V_1 form. The authors concluded that the ventricular myosin isoenzyme pattern is under dominant control of androgens. Since specific receptors for androgens exist in the rat heart (Krieg et al. 1978), and since testosterone treatment enhanced RNA and protein concentrations of the ventricular myocardium (König et al. 1982), the observed effects on the hearts after gonadectomy or gonadectomy and dihydrotestosterone replacement may be explained by the anabolic effects of androgens. Whether the observed effects of dihydrotestosterone on the rat heart are mediated via direct or indirect mechanisms or through modulation at the level of transcription or through posttranscriptional mechanisms cannot be decided yet. In experimentally induced (Lompre et al. 1979) or genetically determined hypertension of male and female rats (Morano et al. 1986; Engelmann et al. 1987), cardiac hypertrophy, and a shift of the myosin isoenzyme pattern to the V_3 form has been consistently observed. A close correlation between cardiac hypertrophy (Rupp and Jacob 1986), systolic blood pressure (Lompre et al. 1979), and ventricular myosin isoenzyme pattern has therefore been proposed. The results of the study of Lengsfeld et al. (1988), however, suggest that androgens dissociate the ventricular myosin isoenzyme pattern from both cardiac hypertrophy and blood pressure. It has been shown (Hoh et al. 1978) that both types of myosin isoforms may respond differently to elevated levels of cyclic AMP caused by β-adrenergic stimulation: cyclic AMP increases V_1 ATPase activity and reduces V_3 ATPase activity. In view of the modulation of the sympathetic nervous system by androgens (Salt 1972; Lara et al. 1985), the change of the myosin isoenzyme pattern induced by dihydrotestosterone in the hearts of the SHRSP may at least partially be explained by its influence on adrenergic transmitter concentration in the synaptic cleft.

2.8 Conclusion

The reports reviewed here suggest that testosterone is a major determinant of the sexual dimorphism with regard to blood pressure and related parameters. There are multiple interactions of testosterone with cardiovascular control mechanisms at several levels of its organization which may contribute to the reported gender differences in cardiovascular function both in physiological and pathophysiological conditions. The reported sex differences in cardiovascular function and the modulating effects of testosterone may well contribute to the higher mortality of men compared to women. On the other hand, the role of estrogens and progesterone which have not been discussed here must also be considered. The impressive sexual dimorphism with regard to blood pressure and the interaction of gonadal steroids with genes which are relevant for cardiovascular control, e.g., the genes coding for components of the renin-angiotensin system, may provide useful model systems for studies directed towards the discovery of the cellular and genetic basis of hypertension.

References

Altura BM (1975) Sex and estrogens and responsiveness of terminal arterioles to neurohypophyseal hormones and catecholamines. J Pharmacol Exp Ther 193:403-412

Ashton N, Balment RJ (1991) Sexual dimorphism in renal function and hormonal status of New Zealand genetically hypertensive rats. Acta Endocrinol (Copenh.) 124:91-97

Bader M, Zhao Y, Sander M, Lee M, Bachmann J, Böhm M, Djavidani B, Peters J, Mullins J, Ganten D (1992) Role of tissue renin in the pathophysiology of hypertension in TGR(mREN2)27. Hypertension, in press

Baker PJ, Ramey PW, Ramwell PW (1978) Androgen-mediated sex differences of cardiovascular responses in rats. Am J Physiol 235:H242-H246

Bardin CW, Catterall JF (1981) Testosterone: a major determinant of extragenital sexual dimorphism. Science 211:1285-1294

Berger FG, Loose D, Meisner H, Watson G (1986) Androgen induction of messenger RNA concentrations in mouse kidney is posttranscriptional. Biochemistry 25:1170-1175

Bhargava KP, Dhavan KN, Saxena RC (1967) Enhancement of noradrenaline pressor responses in testosterone treated cats. Br J Pharmacol 31:26-31

Bonsall RW, Rees HD, Michael RP (1985) The distribution, nuclear uptake and metabolism of [^{3}H]dihydrotestosterone in the brain, pituitary gland and genital tract of the male rhesus monkey. J Steroid Biochem 23:389-394

Brock ML, Shapiro DJ (1983) Estrogen stabilizes vitellogenin mRNA against cytoplasmatic degradation. Cell 34:207-214

Buggy J, Fisher AE (1976) Anteroventral third ventricle site of action for angiotensin induced thirst. Pharmac Biochem Behav 4:651-660

Cambotti LJ, Cole FE, Gerall AA, Frohlich ED, MacPhee AA (1984) Neonatal gonadal hormones and blood pressure in the spontaneously hypertensive rat. Am J Physiol 247:258-264

Carroll JE, Goodfriend TL (1984) Androgen modulation of adrenal angiotensin receptors. Science 224:1009-1011

Christensen LW, Gorski RA (1978) Independent masculinization of neuroendocrine systems by intracerebral implants of testosterone or estradiol in the neonatal female rat. Brain Res 146:325-340

Cirillo M, Trevisan M (1992) The Gubbio Data. Epidemiology and pathophysiology. Clin Exp Hypertens [A] 14:261-269

Clark JH, Schrader WT, O'Malley BT (1985) Mechanisms of steroid hormone action. In: Wilson JD, Foster DW (Eds). W.B. Saunders, Philadelphia, pp 33-75

Cogan MG (1990) Angiotensin II: A powerful controller of sodium transport in the early proximal tubule. Hypertension 15:451-458

Crofton JT, Share L, Shade RE, Lee-Kwon WJ, Manning M, Sawyer WH (1979) The importance of vasopressin in the development and maintenance of DOC-salt hypertension in the rat. Hypertension 1:31-38

Cunard C, Falcon J, Maddox Y, Ridniger M, Ramwell PW (1987) Eicosanoid expression of vascular sexual dimorphism. In: Gryglewski RJ, Stock G (Eds.) Prostacyclin and its stable analogue Ilioprost. Springer Verlag, Berlin, pp 115-122

Daud AI, Bumpus FM, Husain A (1990) Characterization of angiotensin I-converting enzyme (ACE)-containing follicles in the rat ovary during the estrous cycle and effects of ACE inhibitor on ovulation. Endocrinology 126:2927-2935

Dawber TR (1980) The Framingham Study. The Epidemiology of Atherosclerotic Disease. Harvard University Press, Cambridge, MA

Diz DI, Jacobowitz DM (1984) Cardiovascular actions of four neuropeptides in the rat hypothalamus. Clin Exp Hypertens [A] 6:2085-2090

Do YS, Sherrod A, Lobo RA, Paulson RJ, Shinagawa T, Chen S, Kjos S, Hsueh WA (1988) Human ovarian theca cells are a source of renin. Proc Natl Acad Sci USA 85:1957-1961

Dunham EW (1976) Effects of prostaglandins on renal blood flow in the rat. Fed Proc 35:223 (Abstract)

Dunn JF, Nisula BC, Rodbard D (1981) Transport of steroid hormones: binding of 21 endogenous steroids to both testosterone-binding globulin and corticosteroid-binding globulin in human plasma. J Clin Endocrinol Metab 53:58-69

Dzau VJ, Ingelfinger JR (1989) Molecular biology and pathophysiology of the intrarenal renin-angiotensin system. J Hypertens Suppl 7:3-8

Eiff AW, Gogolin E, Jacobs U, Neus H (1986) Ambulatory blood pressure in children followed for 3 years: influence of sex and family history of hypertension. Clin Exp Hypertens [A] 8:577-581

Ellison KE, Ingelfinger JR, Pivor M, Dzau VJ (1989) Androgen regulation of rat renal angiotensinogen messenger RNA expression. J Clin Invest 83:1941-1945

Ely DL, Turner ME (1990) Hypertension in the spontaneously hypertensive rat is linked to the Y chromosome. Hypertension 16:277-281

Engelmann GL, Vitullo JC, Gerrity RG (1987) Morphometric analysis of cardiac hypertrophy during development, maturation, and senescence in spontaneously hypertensive rats. Circ Res 60:487-494

Fischer GM (1972) In vivo effects of estradiol on collagen and elastin dynamics in rat aorta. Endocrinology 91:1227-1232

Fischer GM, Swain ML (1977) Effect of sex hormones on blood pressure and vascular connective tissue in castrated and noncastrated male rats. Am J Physiol 232:H617-H621

Fishman MC, Zimmerman EA, Slater EE (1981) Renin and angiotensin: the complete system within the neuroblastoma x glioma cell. Science 214:921-9923

Fulton R, Birnie GD (1985) Post-transcriptional regulation of rat liver gene expression by glucocorticoids. Nucleic Acids Res 13:6467-6482

Fuxe K, Bunnemann B, Aronsson M, Tinner B, Cintra A, von Euler G, Agnati LF, Nakanishi S, Ohkubo H, Ganten D (1988) Pre- and postsynaptic features of the central angiotensin systems. Indications for a role of angiotensin peptides in volume transmission and for interactions with central monoamine neurons. Clin Exp Hypertens [A] 10:143-168

Ganten D, Fuxe K, Phillips MI, Mann JFE, Ganten U (1978) The brain isorenin-angiotensin system: Biochemistry, localization and possible role in drinking and blood pressure regulation. In: Ganong WF, Martini L (Eds) Frontiers in Neuroendocrinology. Vol.5. Raven Press, New York pp 61-99

Ganten D, Hermann K, Bayer C, Unger Th, Lang RE (1983) Angiotensin synthesis in the brain and increased turnover in hypertensive rats. Science 221:869-871

Ganten D, Lang RE, Lehmann E, Unger T (1984) Brain angiotensin: on the way to becoming a well-studied neuropeptide system. Biochem Pharmacol 33:3523-3528

Ganten D, Lindpaintner K, Ganten U, Peters J, Zimmermann F, Bader M, Mullins J (1991) Transgenic rats: New animal models in hypertension research. Hypertension 17:843-855

Ganten U, Schröder G, Witt M, Zimmermann F, Ganten D, Stock G (1989) Sexual dimorphism of blood pressure in spontaneously hypertensive rats: effects of anti-androgen treatment. J Hypertens 7:721-726

Gomez RA, Lynch KR, Chevalier RL, Everett AD, Johns DW, Wilfong N, Peach MJ, Carey RM (1988) Renin and angiotensinogen gene expression and intrarenal renin distribution during ACE inhibition. Am J Physiol 254:900-906

Greenberg S, George WR, Kadowitz PJ, Wilson WR (1974) Androgen-induced enhancement of vascular reactivity. Can J Physiol Pharmacol 52:14-22

Hackenthal E, Paul M, Ganten D, Taugner R (1990) Morphology, physiology, and molecular biology of renin secretion. Physiol Rev 70:1067-1116

HDFP Cooperative Group (1977) Race, education and prevalence of hypertension. Am J Epidemiol 106:351-361

Hellmann W, Suzuki F, Ohkubo H, Nakanishi S, Ludwig G, Ganten D (1988) Angiotensinogen gene expression in extrahepatic rat tissues: Application of a solution hybridization assay. Naunyn-Schmiedeberg's Arch Pharmacol 338:327-331

Heritage AS, Stumpf WE, Sar M, Grant LD (1980) Brainstem catecholamine neurons as target sites for sex steroid hormones. Science 207:1377-1379

Hoh JFY, McGrath PA, Hale PT (1978) Electrophoretic analysis of multiple forms of rat cardiac myosin: Effect of hypophysectomy and thyroxine replacement. J Mol Cell Cardiol 11:1053-1078

Holm I, Ollo R, Panthier J-J, Rougeon F (1984) Evolution of aspartyl proteases by gene duplication: the mouse renin gene is organized in two homologous clusters of four exons. EMBO J 3:557-562

Iams SG, Wexler BC (1979) Retardation in the development of spontaneous hypertension in SH rats by gonadectomy or estradiol. J Lab Clin Med 94:608-619

Ingelfinger JR, Zuo WM, Fon EA, Ellison KE, Dzau VJ (1990) In situ hybridization evidence for angiotensinogen messenger RNA in the rat proximal tubule. An hypothesis for the intrarenal renin angiotensin system. J Clin Invest 85:417-423

Keil LC, Summy Long J, Severs WB (1975) Release of vasopressin by angiotensin II. Endocrinology 96:1063-1065

Kimura S, Mullins JJ, Bunnemann B, Metzger R, Hilgenfeldt U, Zimmermann F, Jacob H, Fuxe K, Ganten D, Kaling M (1992) High blood pressure in transgenic mice carrying the rat angiotensinogen gene. EMBO J 11:821-827

König H, Goldstone A, Lu CY (1982) Testosterone-mediated sexual dimorphism of the rodent heart. Circ Res 50:782-787

Krieg M, Smith K, Bartsch W (1978) Demonstration of a specific androgen receptor in rat heart muscle. Relationship between binding, metabolism, and tissue level of androgens. Endocrinology 103:1686-1694

Lara H, Galleguillos X, Arran J, Belmar J (1985) Effects of castration and testosterone on norepinephrine storage and on release of [^{3}H]norepinephrine from rat vas deferens. Neurochem Int 7:667-674

Lengsfeld M, Morano I, Ganten U, Ganten D, Rüegg C (1988) Gonadectomy and hormonal replacement changes systolic blood pressure and ventricular myosin isoenzyme pattern of spontaneously hypertensive rats. Circ Res 63:1090-1094

Lindpaintner K, Ganten D (1991) The cardiac renin-angiotensin system - An appraisal of present experimental and clinical evidence. Circ Res 68:905-921

Lindpaintner K, Takahashi S, Ganten D (1990) Structural alterations of the renin gene in stroke-prone spontaneously hypertensive rats: examination of genotype-phenotype correlations. J Hypertens 8:763-773

Lloyd S (1959) The vascular responses of the rat during the reproductive cycle. J Physiol 148:625-632

Lompre AM, Schwartz K, D'Albis A, Lacombe G, Van Thiem N, Swynghedauw B (1979) Myosin isoenzyme redistribution in chronic heart overload. Nature 282:105-117

Malvin RL (1971) Possible role of the renin-angiotensin system in the regulation of antidiuretic hormone secretion. Fed Proc 30:1383-1386

Mangiapane ML, Skoog KM, Rittenhouse P, Blair ML, Sladek CD (1989) Lesions of the area postrema region attenuates hypertension in spontaneously hypertensive rats. Circ Res 64:129-135

Matsudaira T, Kogo H, Satoh T (1985) A possible role of gonad and renal prostaglandin E2 on the development of hypertension in spontaneously hypertensive rats. Jpn J Pharmacol 37:51-57

McEwen BS (1980) Binding and metabolism of sex steroids by the hypothalamic-pituitary unit: physiological implications. Annu Rev Physiol 42:97-115

McEwen BS (1981) Neural gonadal steroid actions. Science 211:1303-1311

McKnight GS, Palmiter RD (1979) Transcriptional regulation of the oval-bumin and conalbumin genes by steroid hormones in chick oviduct. J Biol Chem 254:9050-9058

Metzger R, Wagner D, Takahashi S, Suzuki F, Lindpaintner K, Ganten D (1988) Tissue renin-angiotensin systems: aspects of molecular biology and pharmacology. Clin Exp Hypertens [A] 10:1227-1238

Michael RP, Bonsall RW, Rees HD (1986) The nuclear accumulation of [^{3}H]testosterone and [^{3}H]estradiol in the brain of the female primate: evidence for the aromatization hypothesis. Endocrinology 118:1935-1944

Mooradian AD, Morley JE, Korenman SG (1987) Biological actions of androgens. Endocr Rev 8:1-28

Morano I, Gagelmann M, Arner A, Ganten U, Rüegg JC (1986) Myosin isoenzymes of vascular smooth and cardiac muscle in the spontaneously hypertensive and normotensive male and female rat: a comparative study. Circ Res 59:456-462

Mouw D, Bonjour JP, Malvin RL, Vander A (1971) Central action of angiotensin in stimulating ADH release. Am J Physiol 220:239-242

Mullins JJ, Peters J, Ganten D (1990) Fulminant hypertension in transgenic rats harbouring the mouse Ren-2 gene. Nature 344:541-544

Naruse K, Naruse M, Obana K, Demura R, Demura H, Inagami T, Shizume K (1986) Renin in the rat pituitary coexists with angiotensin and depends on testosterone. Endocrinology 118:2470-2476

Needleman P, Marshall GR, Johnson EM (1974) Determinants and modification of adrenergic and vascular resistance in the kidney. Am J Physiol 227:665-669

Neri R, Kassem N (1984) Biological and clinical properties of anti-androgens. Prog Cancer Res Ther 31:507-518

Neumann F, Hasan SH (1980) Clinical and pharmacological properties of cyproterone acetate: a potent antiandrogen. In: Parvez H, Parvez S (Eds) Advances in Experimental Medicine. Elsevier Biomedical Press, Amsterdam pp 429-476

Neumann F, Kramer M (1966) Female brain differentiation of male rats as a result of early treatment with an androgen antagonist. In: Excerpta Medica Int 1966, Congress Series No. 132 pp 932-941

Neumann F, Steinbeck H (1972) Influence of sexual hormones on the differentiation of neural centers. Arch Sex Behav 2:147-162

Oda H, Lotshaw DP, Franco-Saenz R, Mulrow PJ (1991) Local generation of angiotensin II as a mechanism of aldosterone secretion in rat adrenal capsules. Proc Soc Exp Biol Med 196:175-177

Ohkubo H, Kawakami H, Kakehi Y, Takumi T, Arai H, Yokota Y, Iwai M, Tanabe Y, Masu M, Hata J, Iwao H, Okamoto H, Yokoyama M, Nomura T, Katsuki M, Nakanishi S (1990) Generation of transgenic mice with elevated blood pressure by introduction of the rat renin and angiotensinogen genes. Proc Natl Acad Sci USA 87:5153-5157

Okamura T, Clements DL, Inagami T (1981) Renin, angiotensins, and angiotensin converting enzyme in neuroblastoma cell. Evidence for intracellular formation of angiotensins. Proc Natl Acad Sci USA 78:6940-6943

Oliver WJ, Gross F (1967) Effect of testosterone on submaxillary gland renin-like principle. Am J Physiol 213:341-346

Parmentier M, Inagami T, Pochet R, Desclin JC (1983) Pituitary-dependent renin-like immunoreactivity in the rat testis. Endocrinology 112:1318-1323

Paul M, Bachmann J, Ganten D (1992) The tissue renin-angiotensin systems in cardiovascular disease. Trends Cardiovasc Med 2:94-99

Phoenix CH, Goy RW, Gerall AA, Young WC (1959) Organizing action of prenatally administered testosterone propionate on the tissues mediating mating behavior in the female guinea pig. Endocrinology 65:369-377

Piper PJ, Vane JR (1969) Release of additional factors in anaphylaxis and its antagonism by anti-inflammatory drugs. Nature 223:29-35

Pratt RE, Dzau VJ, Ouellette AJ (1984) Influence of androgen on translatable renin mRNA in the mouse submandibular gland. Hypertension 6:605-613

Pratt RE, Zou WM, Naftilan AJ, Ingelfinger JR, Dzau VJ (1989) Altered sodium regulation of renal angiotensinogen mRNA in the spontaneously hypertensive rat. Am J Physiol 256:H469-H474

Ramsay DJ, Keil LC, Sharpe MC, Shinsako J (1978) Angiotensin II infusion increases vasopressin, ACTH and 11-hydroxycorticosteroid secretion. Am J Physiol 234:R66-R71

Rees HD, Michael RP (1984) Autoradiographic localization of estrogen target cells in the brain, pituitary, and reproductive tract of the male rhesus monkey. Fed Proc 43:913 (Abstract)

Rhees RW, Shryne JE, Gorski RA (1990) Termination of the hormone-sensitive period for differentiation of the sexually dimorphic nucleus of the preoptic area in male and female rats. Brain Res Dev Brain Res 52:17-23

Rupp H, Jacob R (1986) Myocardial transitions between fast- and slow-type muscle as monitored by the population of myosin isoenzymes. In: Rupp H (Eds) Regulation of Heart Function: Basic Concepts and Clinical Applications. Thieme-Verlag, Stuttgart/New York pp 305-326

Salt PJ (1972) Inhibition of noradrenaline uptake in the isolated rat heart by steroids, clonidine and methoxylated phenylethylamines. Eur J Pharmacol 20:329-340

Schaible TF, Malhotra A, Ciambrone G, Scheuer J (1984) The effects of gonadectomy on left ventricular function and cardiac contractile proteins in male and female rats. Circ Res 54:38-49

Schelling P, Fischer H, Ganten D (1991) Angiotensin and cell growth: a link to cardiovascular hypertrophy? J Hypertens 9:3-15

Scheuer J, Malhotra A, Schaible TF, Capasso J (1987) Effects of gonadectomy and hormonal replacement on rat hearts. Circ Res 54:38-49

Schlager G (1968) Genetic and physiological studies of blood pressure in mice. Can J Genet Cytol 10:833-864

Schlager G, Weibust RS (1967) Genetic control of blood pressure in mice. Genetics 55:497-508

Seikaly MG, Arant BS Jr, Seney FD Jr (1990) Endogenous angiotensin concentrations in specific intrarenal fluid compartments of the rat. J Clin Invest 86:1352-1357

Share L, Crofton JT, Ouchi Y (1988) Vasopressin: sexual dimorphism in secretion, cardiovascular actions and hypertension. Am J Med Sci 31:314-319

Skoog KM, Mangiapane ML (1988) Area postrema and cardiovascular regulation in rats. Am J Physiol 254:H963-H969

Slater EE, Defendini R, Zimmerman EA (1980) Wide distribution of immunoreactive renin in nerve cells of human brain. Proc Natl Acad Sci USA 77:5458-5660

St-Louis J, Parent A, Lariviere R, Schiffrin EL (1986) Vasopressin responses and receptors in the mesenteric vasculature of estrogen-treated rats. Am J Physiol 251:H885-H889

Stumpf WE (1990) Steroid hormones and the cardiovascular system: direct actions of estradiol, progesterone, testosterone, gluco- and mineralocorticoids, and soltriol [vitamin D] on central nervous regulatory and peripheral tissues. Experientia 46:13-25

Theveny B, Bailly A, Rauch CM, Delain E, Milgrom E (1987) Association of DNA-bound progesterone receptor. Nature 329:79-81

Tobet SA, Shim JH, Osiecki ST, Baum MJ, Canick JA (1985) Androgen aromatization and 5-alpha reduction in ferret brain during perinatal development: effects of sex and testosterone manipulation. Endocrinology 116:1869-1877

Toscano V (1986) Dihydrotestosterone metabolism. Clin Endocrinol Metab 15:279-292

Tronik D, Rougeon F (1988) Thyroxine and testosterone transcriptionally regulate renin gene expression in the submaxillary gland of normal and transgenic mice carrying extra copies of the Ren2 gene. FEBS Lett 234:336-340

Urata H, Khosla MC, Bumpus FM, Husain A (1988) Evidence for extracellular, but not intracellular, generation of angiotensin II in the rat adrenal zona glomerulosa. Proc Natl Acad Sci USA 85:8251-8255

Uzunova A, Ramey ER, Ramwell PW (1976) Effect of testosterone, sex and age on experimentally induced arterial thrombosis. Nature 261:712-713

Wagner D, Metzger R, Paul M, Ludwig G, Suzuki F, Takahashi S, Murakami K, Ganten D (1990) Androgen dependence and tissue specificity of renin messenger RNA expression in mice. J Hypertens 8:45-52

Wilson CM, Cherry M, Taylor BA, Wilson JD (1981) Genetic and endocrine control of renin activity in the submaxillary gland of the mouse. Biochem Genet 19:509-523

Wilson JD, George FW, Griffin JE (1981) The hormonal control of sexual development. Science 211:1303-1311

Wolinsky H (1972) Effects of androgen treatment on the male rat aorta. J Clin Invest 51:2552-2555

3 Sexual Dimorphism in the Cardiovascular Actions of Vasopressin

Leonard Share and Joan T. Crofton

3.1 Introduction

Vasopressin is synthesized in the magnocellular neurosecretory neurons of the hypothalamic paraventricular and supraoptic nuclei. The hormone is transported along the axons of these neurons to the posterior pituitary gland, where it is stored until it is released into the circulation in response to an appropriate stimulus. The primary physiological stimuli for this release are an increase in plasma osmolality, sensed by osmoreceptors in the brain, and reductions in arterial blood pressure or blood volume, sensed by the arterial baroreceptors and cardiac receptors. Afferents from these cardiovascular receptors ascend to centers in the medulla involved in cardiovascular regulation. Pathways from these centers project to the paraventricular and supraoptic nuclei. The neural control of vasopressin release has been reviewed recently (e.g., Bisset and Chowdrey 1988; Renaud and Bourque 1991). Estrogen and androgen receptors are found in centers in the brain involved in the control of vasopressin secretion and in cardiovascular regulation (Stumpf and Sar 1977; Heritage et al. 1980), suggesting that the gonadal steroid hormones can act centrally to modulate these functions.

Vasopressin is well known as the antidiuretic hormone, promoting water reabsorption by the kidney. Vasopressin is also an extremely potent vasoconstrictor, perhaps more potent than angiotensin II (Altura and Altura 1977). Vasopressin at plasma concentrations that are physiologically relevant also reduces cardiac output and heart rate (Montani et al. 1980). Thus, the ability of vasopressin to increase blood pressure is the resultant of the reduction in cardiac output and increase in total peripheral resistance.

3.2 Sexual Dimorphism in Vasopressin Secretion

Several years ago we obtained evidence suggesting that the gonadal steroid hormones could affect the release of vasopressin. In humans on a normal sodium diet, the 24-h urinary excretion of vasopressin, an integrated index of vasopressin secretion, was higher in men than in women and higher in blacks than in whites, and there was a similar pattern in plasma vasopressin concentrations (Fig. 1; Crofton et al. 1986a). These differences were probably attenuated, since some of the women were postmenopausal. In rats, the plasma vasopressin concentration was also higher in males than in females (Fig. 2; Crofton et al. 1985). Gonadectomy tended to decrease the plasma vasopressin concentration in males and increase it in females. These effects were reversed by treatment of the male rats with testosterone and the females with progesterone or progesterone plus estrogen (Fig. 2). Since the gender difference in the plasma vasopressin concentration in the rat could not be explained by a difference in the metabolic clearance of vasopressin (Crofton et al. 1986b), it is likely that this difference is due to an action of the gonadal steroid hormones on a central component in the control of vasopressin release. Indeed, in postmenopausal women, the plasma vasopressin concentration was decreased by treatment with estrogen and increased by treatment with both estrogen and proges-

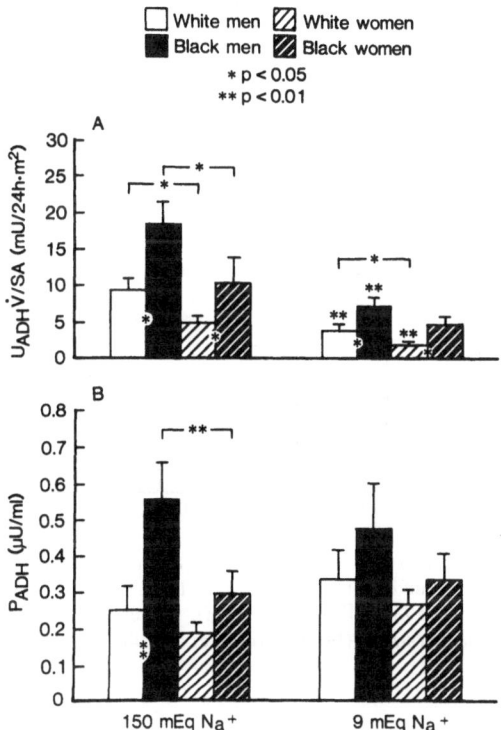

Fig. 1. A The 24-h urinary excretion of vasopressin corrected for body surface area ($U_{ADH}\dot{V}/SA$) and **B** the plasma vasopressin concentration (P_{ADH}) in normal black and white men and women on a normal-sodium diet (150 mmol/day) and a low- sodium diet (9 mmol/day). *Asterisks between the bars* designate significant differences between those groups; *asterisks directly above the bars* designate differences between the normal- and low-sodium diets. (From Crofton et al. 1986a)

togen (Forsling et al. 1982). Whether plasma vasopressin levels change during the course of the menstrual cycle is, however, controversial (Forsling et al. 1981; Punnonen et al. 1983).

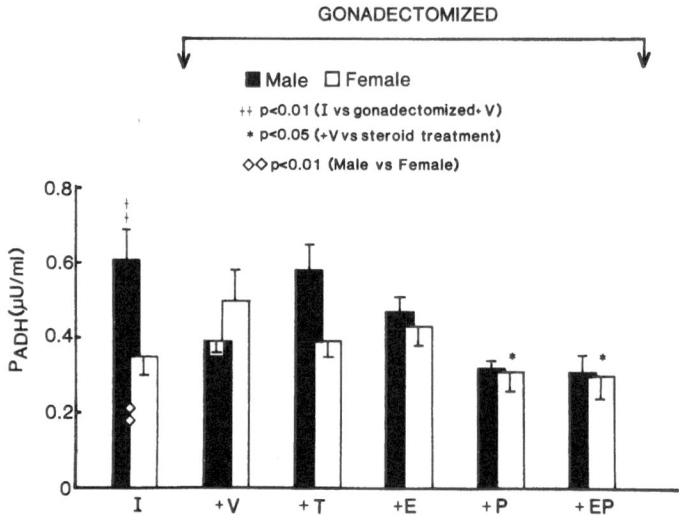

Fig. 2. The plasma vasopressin concentration (P_{ADH}) in intact (*I*) male and female rats and in gonadectomized male and female rats treated with vehicle (*+V*), testosterone (*+T*), 17β-estradiol (*+E*), progesterone (*+P*), and progesterone plus estradiol (*+EP*). (From Crofton et al. 1985)

3.3 Sexual Dimorphism in the Pressor Action of Vasopressin

In the course of determining the metabolic clearance rate of vasopressin by infusing vasopressin i.v. at graded doses, we found that the pressor response to this hormone was greater in male rats than in randomly cycling females (Crofton et al. 1986b). In order to examine this difference more thoroughly, conscious unrestrained male rats and females in each phase of the estrus cycle were given graded i.v. infusion of vasopressin, 30 min at each rate of infusion (Crofton et al. 1988). Mean arterial blood pressure (MABP) was averaged over the last 5 min of each infusion and a blood sample for the measurement of the plasma vasopressin concentration was taken at the end of each infusion. Sampled blood was replaced with rat donor blood. Plasma vasopressin levels were increased to approximately 6 μU/ml (1 μU = 2.5 pg) at the lowest vasopressin infusion and to 40 μU/ml at the highest infusion.

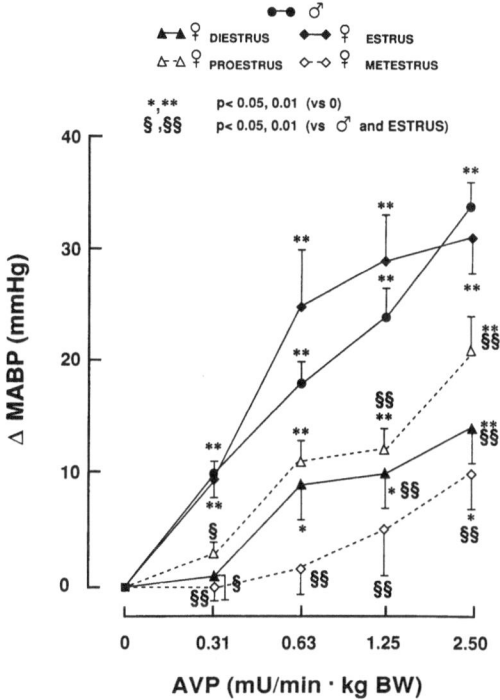

Fig. 3. Changes in mean arterial blood pressure (*ΔMABP*) in response to graded i.v. infusions of vasopressin (*AVP*) in male rats and in female rats in each phase of the estrus cycle. (From Crofton et al. 1988)

The preinfusion plasma vasopressin concentration was higher in males than in the females in each of the phases of the estrus cycle. This difference was small relative to the increases produced by the vasopressin infusions, and there were no significant differences in plasma vasopressin levels with respect to either sex or phase of the estrus cycle at the end of each of the vasopressin infusions.

In male rats and estrus females, there were progressive, virtually identical increases in MABP in response to the graded infusion of vasopressin (Fig. 3). The pressor responses to vasopressin in females in diestrus, proestrus, and metestrus, however, were markedly attenuated

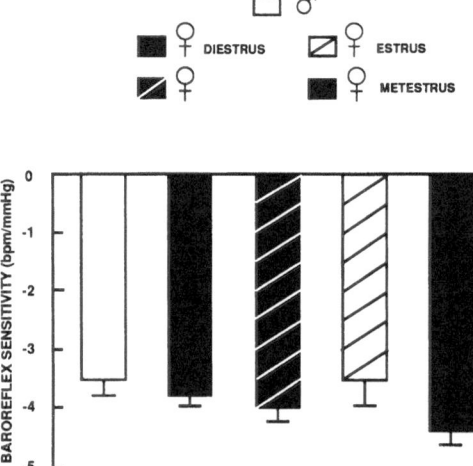

Fig. 4. Baroreflex sensitivity in male rats and in female rats in each phase of the estrus cycle. (From Crofton et al. 1988)

compared to the responses in males and estrus females. This sexually dimorphic pressor response was specific for vasopressin, since we were unable to demonstrate any differences with respect to gender or phase of the estrus cycle in the pressor responses to either angiotensin II or phenylephrine (Crofton et al. 1988).

In order to determine whether the sexually dimorphic pressor response to vasopressin was due to gender effects on the function of the baroreceptor reflex, we evaluated the sensitivity of the cardiac component of the baroreceptor reflex by calculating the slope of the relationship between changes in MABP and heart rate in response to alternating graded bolus i.v. injections of phenylephrine, to increase MABP and reflexly decrease heart rate, and sodium nitroprusside, to decrease MABP and reflexly increase heart rate (Crofton et al. 1988). The slope of this relationship was identical in males and in females in each of the phases of the estrus cycle (Fig. 4).

Although it has been convincingly demonstrated that vasopressin can increase the sensitivity of the baroreceptor reflex in some species, the situation in the rat is controversial (see review by Share 1988). In

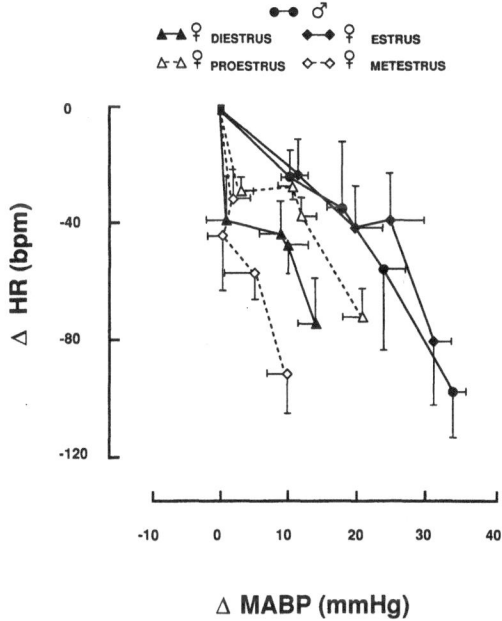

Fig. 5. Relationship between change in mean arterial blood pressure (*ΔMABP*) and change in heart rate (*ΔHR*) in response to graded i.v. infusions of vasopressin in male rats and in female rats in each phase of the estrus cycle. (From Crofton et al. 1988)

view of this, we examined the relationship between the increases in MABP and decreases in heart rate produced by vasopressin in male and female rats (Fig. 5). The slope of this relationship in males and estrus females was similar to that obtained when MABP was altered by nitroprusside and phenylephrine, i.e., vasopressin in these animals had no apparent effect on baroreflex sensitivity. In females in diestrus, proestrus, and metestrus, however, low vasopressin infusion rates caused a marked bradycardia with little or no increase in MABP (this relationship was so nonlinear that slopes could not be calculated), suggesting that, in these groups of rats, vasopressin caused an increased sensitivity of the baroreceptor reflex that could have contributed to the attenuated pressor response to this hormone. The presence of estrogen

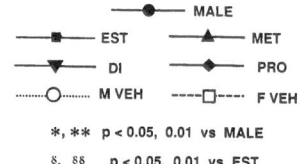

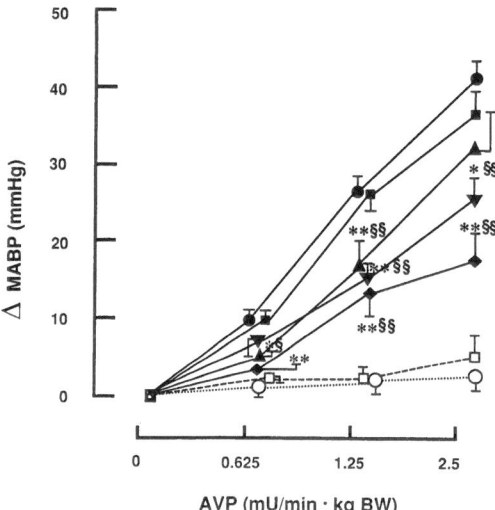

Fig. 6. Changes in mean arterial blood pressure (Δ*MABP*) in response to graded i.v. infusions of vasopressin (*AVP*) in male rats and in estrus (*EST*), diestrus (*DI*), metestrus (*MET*), and proestrus (*PRO*) female rats. Only the saline vehicle for vasopressin was infused in *M VEH* (males) and *F VEH* (randomly cycling females). (From Toba et al. 1991)

and androgen receptors in centers in the brainstem involved in cardiovascular regulation (Heritage et al. 1980) is consistent with this possibility.

It has been demonstrated that vasopressin can stimulate the synthesis of prostaglandins in cultured vascular smooth muscle (Hassid and Williams 1983). It has also been reported that inhibition of prostaglandin synthesis potentiated the pressor response to vasopressin in male rats (Walker et al. 1988). We therefore considered the possibility that the sexually dimorphic pressor response to vasopressin was due to gender-related differences in the stimulation of vascular vasodilator prostaglandins by vasopressin. This was not the case. Pretreatment with indomethacin (5 mg/kg) failed to affect the pressor responses to vasopressin in both male and nonestrus female rats (unpublished observations).

Vasopressin is not only a potent vasoconstrictor, it also decreases cardiac output. Consequently, the sexually dimorphic pressor response to vasopressin could be due to either its vascular or cardiac actions. To resolve this issue, experiments were carried out in conscious male and female rats that were chronically instrumented with arterial and venous catheters and a thermocouple probe in the thoracic aorta for the measurement of cardiac output by the thermal dilution method (Toba et al. 1991). As we had demonstrated previously, the graded i.v. infusion of vasopressin, 40 min at each dose, resulted in greater increases in MABP in male and estrus female rats than in females in the other phases of the estrus cycle (Fig. 6). There were, however, no significant gender- or cycle-related differences in the vasopressin-induced reductions in cardiac output (Fig. 7). Consequently, the sexually dimorphic pressor response was due entirely to differences in the ability of vasopressin to increase total peripheral resistance.

In order to determine the role of the gonadal steroid hormones in this response, the experiments were repeated in gonadectomized rats, some of which were given steroid replacement treatment (Toba et al. 1991). Rats were gonadectomized when they were 3 weeks old, replacement therapy with subcutaneously implanted slow-release steroid-containing pellets was begun 2 weeks later, and the experiments were performed 3-4 weeks after that. Castration in male rats had no effect on the pressor responsiveness to vasopressin (Fig. 8). On the other hand, ovariectomy increased pressor responsiveness to vasopressin to levels seen in males. This effect was reversed by chronic treatment with 17β-estradiol, whereas chronic treatment with progesterone was without effect. The implants of 17β-estradiol and progesterone were estimated to provide plasma concentrations of 100-200 pg/ml and approximately 6 ng/ml, respectively. Since none of the treatments had a significant effect on cardiac output, the effects of ovariectomy and estrogen treatment on the ability of vasopressin to increase MABP were due to differences in increases in total peripheral resistance. Thus,

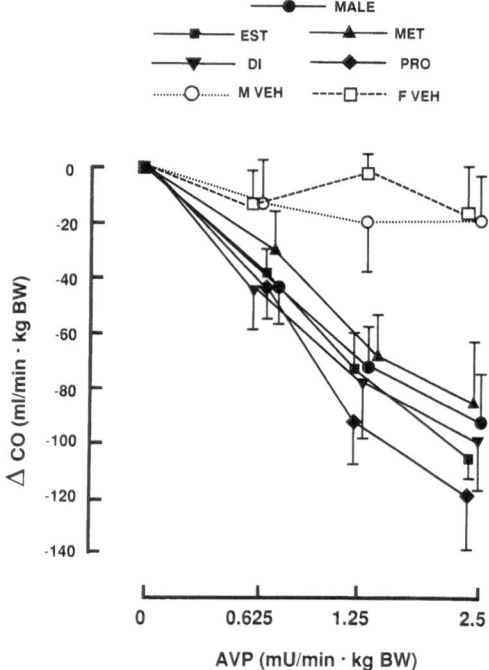

Fig. 7. Changes in cardiac output (ΔCO) in response to graded i.v. infusions of vasopressin (*AVP*) in male rats and in estrus (*EST*), diestrus (*DI*), metestrus (*MET*), and proestrus (*PRO*) female rats. Only the saline vehicle for vasopressin was infused in *M VEH* (males) and *F VEH* (randomly cycling females). (From Toba et al. 1991)

these data suggest that estrogen can attenuate the overall vasoconstrictor response to vasopressin.

There are, however, observations that conflict with this view. Altura (1975) examined the effects of gender and estrogen treatment on the vasoconstrictor responses of microscopically visualized mesenteric arterioles in situ. The dose-response curve for topically applied vasopressin in females was located to the left of that in males, i.e., vasopressin exerted a greater vasoconstrictor action in males than in females. In male rats, pretreatment with a single dose of 17β-estradiol

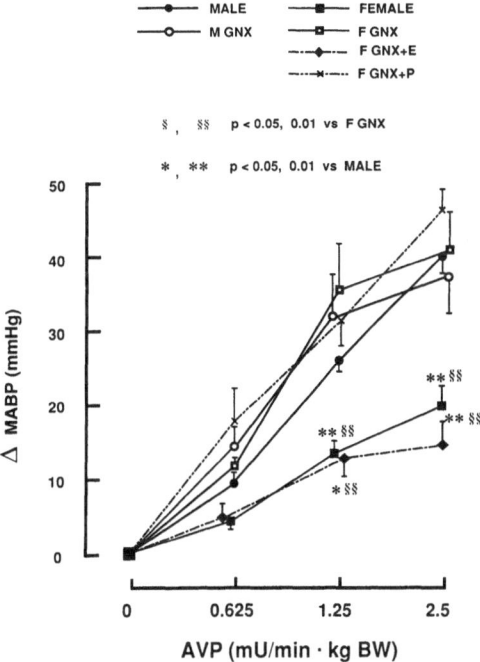

Fig. 8. Changes in mean arterial blood pressure ($\Delta MABP$) in response to graded i.v. infusions of vasopressin in intact male and nonestrus female rats and in gonadectomized males (*M GNX*), gonadectomized females (*F GNX*), gonadectomized females treated with 17β-estradiol (*F GNX+E*), and gonadectomized females treated with progesterone (*F GNX+P*). (From Toba et al. 1991)

increased the vasoconstrictor potency of vasopressin. However, because these experiments were carried out in anesthetized, surgically prepared rats, circulating levels of vasopressin and other vasoconstrictors, e.g., angiotensin II and catecholamines, are likely to have been greatly elevated and could have influenced the response to topically applied vasopressin.

St-Louis et al. (1986) avoided this problem by using the isolated perfused rat mesenteric vascular bed. Treatment with estradiol increased the vasoconstrictor response to vasopressin in ovariectomized females and in intact males. There was, however, no comparison be-

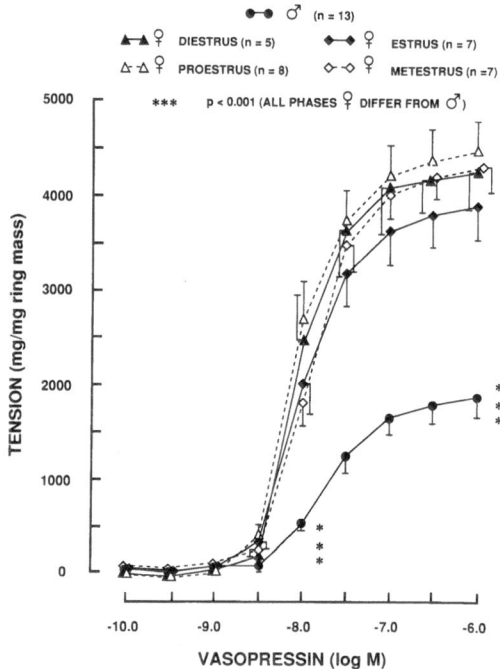

Fig. 9. Concentration-response curves for vasopressin for thoracic aortic rings from male rats and diestrus, proestrus, estrus, and metestrus female rats. Contractile tension is normalized by the dry weight of the aortic rings. (From Stallone et al. 1991)

tween untreated intact males and females. We, therefore, used isolated rat thoracic aortic rings from male rats and from females in each phase of the estrous cycle (Stallone et al. 1991). In contrast to our findings in the intact animal, the vasoconstrictor response to vasopressin was much greater in aortic rings from females than from males, and there were no differences with respect to the phase of the estrus cycle (Fig. 9).

Thus, the experimental findings indicate that estrogen can potentiate the ability of vasopressin to increase total peripheral resistance in vivo, whereas the opposite obtains for the mesenteric vascular bed in vivo and in vitro and the thoracic aorta in vitro. However, the aorta is not a resistance vessel, and the mesenteric circulation is not the primary contributor to total peripheral resistance. These observations suggest, rather, that there is heterogeneity in blood vessels with respect to the ability of estrogen to modulate the vasoconstrictor action of vasopressin and, possibly, other vasoconstrictors as well. Be that as it may, it is apparent that the gonadal steroid hormones, particularly estrogen, contribute importantly to cardiovascular regulation. These hormones could exert this action at the level of the central nervous system and blood vessels, since receptors for the gonadal steroid hormones have been found in these structures (Colbum and Buonassisi; Heritage et al. 1980; Horwitz and Horwitz 1982; Stumpf and Sar 1977). In the brain, these receptors are located in centers involved in cardiovascular regulation (Heritage et al. 1980) and in the control of neurohypophysial hormone synthesis and release (Stumpf and Sar 1977). In blood vessels, it remains to be determined whether estrogen modulates the contractile response to vasopressin via an action on the endothelium or directly on vascular smooth muscle. Although receptors for androgen and estrogen have been found in the heart (Krieg et al. 1978; Stumpf et al. 1977), we were unable to find any evidence for an effect of the gonadal steroid hormones on the cardiac actions of vasopressin (Toba et al. 1991). It is, however, possible that these hormones could exert other actions on cardiac performance.

Hemorrhage is an extremely potent stimulus for vasopressin secretion. When rats were subjected to stepwise hemorrhage, there was no gender difference in their ability to maintain MABP, but stimulation of vasopressin release was greater in nonestrus females than in males (Crofton et al. 1990). Pretreatment with a V_1-receptor antagonist had no effect on the ability of male rats to maintain MABP in the face of the hemorrhage, but blood pressure compensation in females was impaired (Crofton et al. 1990). It appears that vasopressin is particularly important for blood pressure compensation in response to hemorrhage in female rats.

3.4 Sexual Dimorphism in the Antidiuretic Action of Vasopressin

Rats were hydrated and anesthetized with oral doses of water and ethanol; hydration and anesthesia were maintained by the i.v. infusion of a hypotonic saline-dextrose-ethanol solution. Catheters were placed in a jugular vein for infusion, in the abdominal aorta via a femoral artery for measuring MABP, and in the urinary bladder for the collection of urine. In control animals, the rate of urine flow remained relatively constant for the 2-h duration of the experiment. The i.v. infusion of vasopressin at a rate of 20 μU/min/kg body weight resulted in a reduction in urine flow that was significantly greater in males and estrous females than in females in the other phases of the estrus cycle. When vasopressin was infused at a rate of 200 μU/min/kg body weight, the pattern of the responses was similar, but the differences with respect to gender and phase of the estrous cycle were no longer statistically significant. These differences were not due to differences in the plasma concentrations of vasopressin achieved by the infusions, and these doses of vasopressin did not affect MABP.

A possible mechanism for this sexually dimorphic response is suggested by the report by Hatano et al. (1988) that both estradiol and progesterone reduced the stimulation of cAMP generation by vasopressin in cultured renal medullary cells. Increased distal nephron cAMP is involved in the ability of vasopressin to cause an antidiuresis.

The impact of the modulation of the antidiuretic action of vasopressin by the gonadal steroid hormones on water and electrolyte homeostasis and cardiovascular function remains to be determined. In any event, it is noteworthy that both the pressor and the antidiuretic responses to vasopressin are greater in males and in females in estrus than in females in the other phases of the estrus cycle; both estrogen and progesterone are at their lowest during estrus.

3.5 Sexual Dimorphism
in Deoxycorticosterone-Salt Hypertension

Deoxycorticosterone (DOC)-salt hypertension in the rat, which is produced by removing one kidney, treating the rat chronically with DOC, and substituting saline for drinking water, is dependent upon vasopressin. Vasopressin secretion is elevated (Möhring et al. 1977; Crofton et al. 1979), treatment with a V_1-receptor antagonist (Crofton et al. 1979) or a vasopressin antiserum (Möhring et al. 1977) lowers blood pressure, and this model of hypertension cannot be produced in rats with a hereditary inability to synthesize vasopressin (Crofton et al.

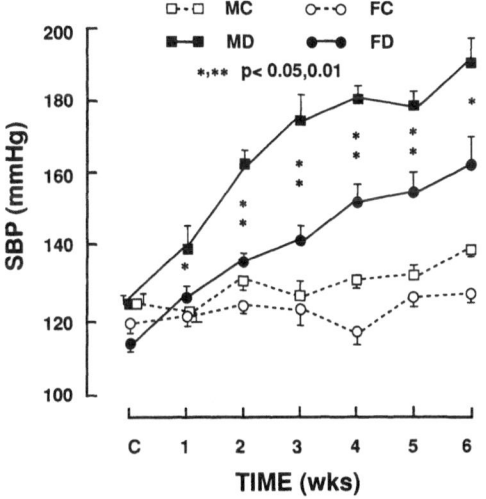

Fig. 10. Systolic blood pressure (*SBP*) of control male (*MC*) and female (*FC*) rats and male (*MD*) and female (*FD*) rats treated with DOC and given 1% saline to drink. (From Ouchi et al. 1987)

1979). The role of vasopressin in DOC-salt hypertension is uncertain, but the data suggest that vasopressin may participate initially as an antidiuretic agent, helping to expand blood volume, and thereby possibly contributing to the development of the hypertension. Subsequently vasopressin contributes as a pressor agent, helping to maintain the elevated blood pressure.

Because of this and because of the greater pressor and antidiuretic responsiveness to vasopressin in male rats than in females in three of the four phases of the estrous cycle, we wondered whether there might be a gender difference in the development of DOC-salt hypertension. This is indeed the case. Blood pressure rises more rapidly and reaches a higher level in male than in female rats (Fig.10; Ouchi et al. 1987). This difference is substantial, approximately 20-30 mmHg during the last several weeks of observation. Vasopressin secretion was elevated in the hypertensive animals, but to a similar extent in the males and females (Ouchi et al. 1987). Pressor responsiveness to vasopressin was greater in the hypertensive males than in the hypertensive females; the

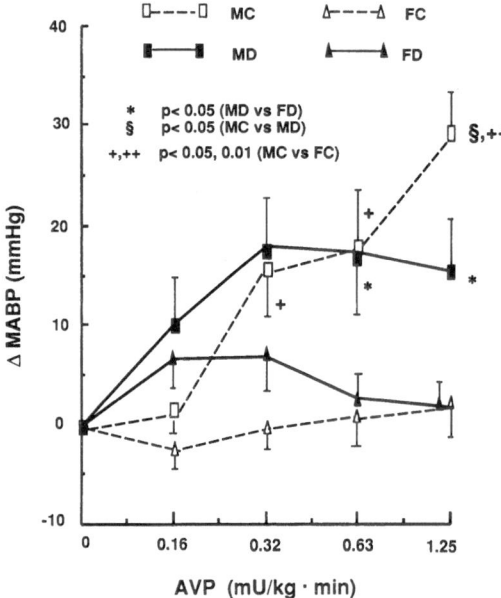

Fig. 11. Changes in mean arterial blood pressure ($\Delta MABP$) in response to graded i.v. infusions of vasopressin (*AVP*) in male control (*MC*), male DOC-salt hypertensive (*MD*), female control (*FC*), and female DOC-salt hypertensive (*FD*) rats 3 weeks after the start of treatment. (From Ouchi et al. 1988)

magnitude of this difference was similar to that observed in normotensive animals (Fig. 11; Ouchi et al. 1988).

As had been reported previously by Matsuguchi and Schmid (1982), baroreflex sensitivity, assessed by the slope of the relationship between change in MABP and change in heart rate in response to alternating graded i.v. injections of phenylephrine and sodium nitroprusside, was attenuated in the hypertensive rats. The magnitude of this attenuation, however, was greater in males than in females (Fig. 12; Ouchi et al. 1988).

We suggest, then, that the gender difference in the development and maintenance of DOC-salt hypertension in the rat is due to several factors. These include the greater pressor and antidiuretic responsiveness to vasopressin in males than in females in most phases of the estrus

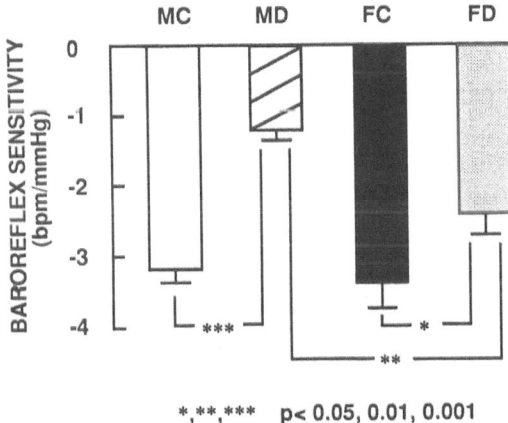

Fig. 12. Baroreflex sensitivity in male control (*MC*), male DOC-salt hypertensive (*MD*), female control (*FC*), and female DOC-salt hypertensive (*FD*) rats 3 weeks after the start of treatment. (Ouchi et al. 1988)

cycle, the elevated plasma levels of vasopressin, and the greater attenuation of the sensitivity of the baroreceptor reflex in males than in females. Other, as yet unidentified factors may also be involved.

We have recently carried out experiments to characterize the role of the gonadal steroid hormones in the sexually dimorphic development of DOC-salt hypertension. Rats were gonadectomized or sham-operated when they were 3 weeks old. At age 5-6 weeks, they were unilaterally nephrectomized and chronic treatment with subcutaneously implanted slowrelease hormone pellets was begun. Treatment with DOC and saline was begun 1 week later. The development and level of the hypertension were attenuated in castrated males and exacerbated in ovariectomized females (Fig. 13; Crofton et al. 1989). These effects were reversed by treating the castrated males with testosterone and the ovariectomized females with 17β-estradiol (unpublished observations). Treatment of the ovariectomized females with progesterone had no effect on the course of the hypertension. When a combination of progesterone and estradiol was used in the ovariectomized rats, the protective action of the estradiol was prevented for the first 2 weeks of the 3-week period of observation; in the 3rd week blood pressure fell to le-

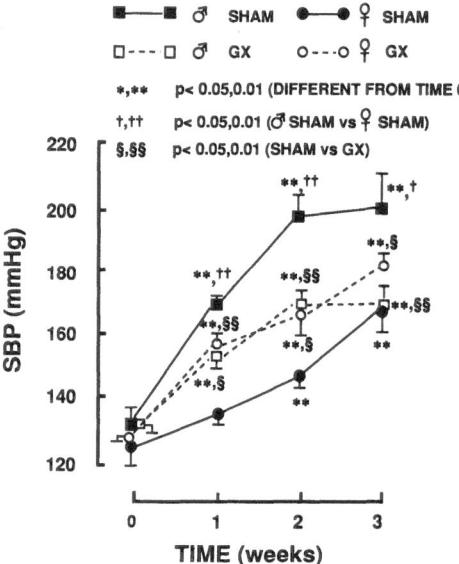

Fig. 13. Systolic blood pressure (*SBP*) in sham-operated (*SHAM*) and gona-dectomized (*GX*) male and female rats made hypertensive by treatment with DOC and substitution of 1% saline for drinking water. (Crofton et al. 1989)

vels seen in the intact females. The development of the hypertension was reduced by treating intact males chronically with 17β-estradiol, whereas treating intact females with testosterone had no effect on the course of the hypertension.

Thus, DOC-salt hypertension is attenuated by estrogen in male and female rats, whereas testosterone exacerbates the hypertension in males and is without effect in females. In females, progesterone temporarily masks the effect of estradiol. The mechanisms underlying these actions of the gonadal steroid hormones are not known, but are likely to involve modulation of the cardiovascular and renal actions of vasopressin. The gonadal steroid hormones could act in the central nervous system, as well as in the peripheral vasculature and the kidney.

3.6 Conclusion

It is, then, apparent that the gonadal steroid hormones participate significantly in cardiovascular regulation. It is likely that this role for these hormones involves, at least in part, modulation of the biological actions of vasopressin.

Acknowledgement. Original research was supported by National Heart, Lung, and Blood Institute grants HL-12990 and HL-19209.

References

Altura BM (1975) Sex and estrogens and responsiveness of terminal arterioles to neurohypophyseal hormones and catecholamines. J Pharmacol Exp Ther 193:403-412

Altura BM, Altura BT (1977) Vascular smooth muscle and neurohypophyseal hormones. Fed Proc 36:1853-1860

Bisset GW, Chowdrey HS (1988) Control of release of vasopressin by neuroendocrine reflexes. J Exp Physiol 73: 811-872

Colburn P, Buonassisi V (1978) Estrogen-binding sites in endothelial cell cultures. Science 201:817-819

Crofton JT, Share L (1989) Sexual dimorphism in vasopressin and cardiovascular response to hemorrhage in the rat. Circ Res 66:1345-1353

Crofton JT, Share L, Shade RE, Lee-Kwon Wj, Manning M, Sawyer WH (1979) The importance of vasopressin in the development and maintenance of DOC-salt hypertension in the rat. Hypertension 1:31-38

Crofton JT, Baer PG, Share L, Brooks DP (1985) Vasopressin release in male and female rats: effects of gonadectomy and treatment with gonadal steroid hormones. Endocrinology 117:1195-1200

Crofton JT, Dustan H, Share L, Brooks DP (1986a) Vasopressin secretion in normotensive black and white men and women on normal and low sodium diets. J Endocrinol 108:191-199

Crofton JT, Ratliff DL, Brooks DP, Share L (1986b) The metabolic clearance rate of and pressor responses to vasopressin in male and female rats. Endocrinology 118:1777-1781

Crofton JT, Share L, Brooks DP (1988) Pressor responsiveness to and secretion of vasopressin during the estrous cycle. Am J Physiol 255:R1041-R1048

Crofton JT, Share L, Brooks DP (1989) Gonadectomy abolishes the sexual dimorphism in DOC-salt hypertension in the rat. Clin Exp Hypertens [A] 11:1249-1261

Forsling ML, Akerlund M, Strbmberg (1981) Variations in plasma concentrations of vasopressin during the menstrual cycle. J Endocrinol 89:263-266

Forsling ML, Strómberg P, Akerlund M (1982) Effect of ovarian steroids on vasopressin secretion. J Endocrinol 95:147-151

Hassid A, Williams C (1983) Vasoconstrictor-evoked prostaglandin synthesis in cultured vascular smooth muscle. Am J Physiol 245:C278-C282

Hatano T, Ogawa K, Kanda K, Seo H, Matsui N (1988) Effect of ovarian steroids on cyclic adenosine 3':5'-monophosphate production stimulated by arginine vasopressin in rat renal monolayer cultured cells. Endocrinol Jpn 35:267-274

Heritage AS, Stumpf WE, Sar M, Grant LD (1980) Brainstem catecholamine neurons are target sites for sex steroid hormones. Science 207:1377-1379

Horwitz KB, Horwitz LD (1982) Canine vascular tissues are targets for androgens, progestins, and glucocorticoids. J Clin Invest 69:750-758

Krieg M, Smith K, Bartsch W (1978) Demonstration of a specific androgen receptor in rat heart muscle: relationship between binding, metabolism, and tissue levels of androgens. Endocrinology 103:1686-1694

Matsuguchi H, Schmid PG (1982) Pressor response to vasopressin and impaired baroreflex function in DOC-salt hypertension. Am J Physiol 242:H44-H49

Möhring J, Möhring B, Petri M, Haack D (1977) Vasopressor role of ADH in the pathogenesis of malignant DOC hypertension. Am J Physiol 232:F260-F269

Montani J-P, Liard J-F, Schoun J, Möhring J (1980) Hemodynamic effects of exogenous and endogenous vasopressin at low plasma concentrations in conscious dogs. Circ Res 17: 346-355

Ouchi Y, Share L, Crofton JT, Iitake K, Brooks DP (1987) Sex difference in the development of deoxycorticosterone-salt hypertension in the rat. Hypertension 9:172-177

Ouchi Y, Share L, Crofton JT, Iitake K, Brooks DP (1988) Sex difference in pressor responsiveness to vasopressin and baroreflex function in DOC-salt hypertensive rats. J Hypertens 6:381-387

Punnonen R, Viinamäki O, Multamäki S (1983) Plasma vasopressin during normal menstrual cycle. Hormone Res 17:90-92

Renaud LP, Bourque CW (1991) Neurophysiology and neuropharmacology of hypothalamic magnocellular neurons secreting vasopressin and oxytocin. Prog Neurobiol 36:131-169

Share L (1988) Role of vasopressin in cardiovascular regulation. Physiol Rev 68:1248-1283

Stallone JN, Crofton JT, Share L (1991) Sexual dimorphism in vasopressin-induced contraction of rat aorta. Am J Physiol 260:H453-H458

St-Louis J, Parent A, Larivière R, Schiffrin EL (1986) Vasopressin responses and receptors in the mesenteric vasculature of estrogen treated rats. Am J Physiol 251:H885-H889

Stumpf WE (1990) Steroid hormones and the cardiovascular system: direct actions of estradiol, progesterone, testosterone, gluco- and mineralcorticoids, and soltriol [vitamin D] on central nervous regulatory and peripheral tissues. Experientia 46:13-25

Stumpf WE, Sar M (1977) Steroid hormone target cells in the periventricular brain: relationship to peptide hormone producing cells. Fed Proc 36:1973-1977

Stumpf WE, Sar M (1977) The heart: a target organ for estradiol. Science 196:319-321

Toba K, Crofton JT, Inoue M, Share L (1991) Effects of vasopressin on arterial blood pressure and cardiac output in male and female rats. Am J Physiol 261:R1118-R1125

Walker BR, Brizzee BL, Harrison-Bernard LM (1988) Potentiated vasoconstrictor response to vasopressin following meclofenamate in conscious rats (42649). Proc Soc Exp Biol Med 187:157-164

4 Cardiovascular Adaptation to Pregnancy

Mark J. Morton

4.1 Introduction

Traditional descriptions of the cardiovascular adjustments to pregnancy are dominated by the elevated blood volume and reduced resistance in the uteroplacental circulation. Other mechanisms followed logically from the plethora and reduced vascular resistance. Studies of the timing of hemodynamic changes during pregnancy and of the adaptation of the heart, arteries and venous capacitance beds suggest that extensive changes in the circulation occur early in pregnancy which may be independent of blood volume and uterine vascular resistance changes. At least some of the changes characteristic of pregnancy can be produced by sex steroids and therefore may be hormonally mediated.

4.2 Blood Volume

Blood volume increases are consistently found in all mammalian species studied. In the human, blood volume increases 40–50% above control levels with a peak in the middle of the third trimester (Hytten and Paintin 1963). The increase in blood volume is linear and appears to be related to the total fetal mass. Blood volume varies with the size of the fetus and number of fetuses (Letsky 1980). Total hemoglobin is increased during pregnancy, but not in proportion to the increase in blood volume, because of a relatively larger increase in plasma volume. This results in the "physiologic anemia of pregnancy." Longo (1983) proposed that maternal blood volume is regulated by the fetus and placenta through a feedback mechanism in order to optimize fetal development. Estrogen substrate, dehydroepiandrosterone, is produced by the fetal adrenal gland. In the maternal circulation, the estrogens stimulate the production of renin eventually resulting in increased aldosterone. Plasma volume is then increased because of salt and water absorption. Other hormones are responsible for facilitating the increase in total hemoglobin.

4.3 Cardiac Output

4.3.1 Magnitude and Timing of Changes

As with blood volume, all mammalian species that have been studied have cardiac output increases during pregnancy. Cardiac output is an inherently labile parameter and, until recently, invasive methods were necessary for accurate assessment. In human pregnancy the uterus is large enough in the third trimester to obstruct inferior vena cava flow and thus limit venous return in most postures (Ueland et al. 1969; Kerr

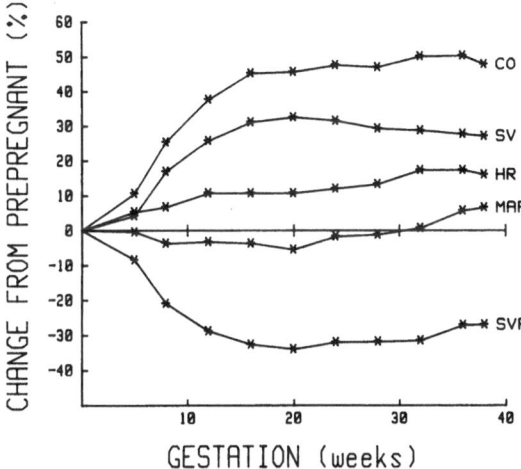

Fig. 1. The data from 13 women studied serially by Robson et al. (1989) before and during pregnancy are shown as percent change from prepregnant for: *CO*, cardiac output, *SV*, stroke volume, *HR*, heart rate, *MAP*, mean arterial pressure, *SVR*, systemic vascular resistance. Flow was calculated from aortic velocity and cross-sectional area. (From Morton 1990)

et al. 1964). Recently, Robson et al. (1989) completed a serial, prospective study of hemodynamics during human pregnancy utilizing Doppler and cross-sectional echocardiography. Results derived from the estimates of aortic flow throughout pregnancy are shown in Fig. 1. Cardiac output increases rapidly to 40–50% above control levels early in the second trimester of pregnancy and reaches a plateau after this time. Stroke volume also reaches a peak in the second trimester and may decline slightly before delivery. Heart rate increases progressively throughout gestation. Arterial pressure reaches a nadir in the middle of the second trimester and then returns to control values at the end of gestation. Because of the marked increase in cardiac output and a slight fall in mean arterial pressure, vascular resistance reaches its nadir in the middle of the second trimester.

The magnitude and timing of these changes are important for two reasons. First, they aid clinicians in the care of patients who have coexistent pregnancy and cardiovascular disease. Second, the timing of

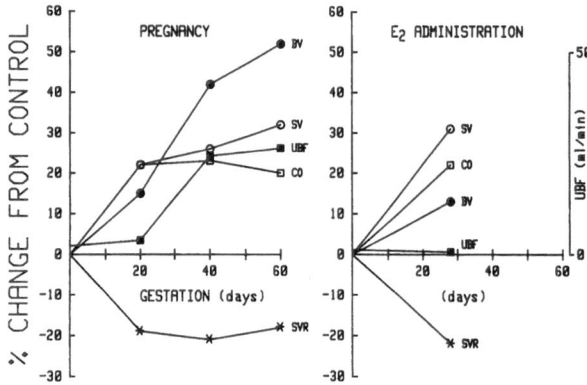

Fig. 2. The data from pregnant and estrogen treated guinea pigs are shown as percent change from matched controls throughout pregnancy or 28 days of estradiol administration. *BV,* blood volume, *SV,* stroke volume, *UBF,* uterine blood flow, *CO,* cardiac output, *SVR,* systemic vascular resistance. (Modified from Hart et al. 1985)

changes can be used to increase understanding of the physiology of cardiovascular adaptations to pregnancy. From the previous description, it is obvious that the blood volume changes characteristic of pregnancy do not coincide with the marked increases in stroke volume and cardiac output early in pregnancy. Likewise, the increase in uterine blood flow during human pregnancy is out of phase with the increase in cardiac output (Assali et al. 1960; Metcalfe et al. 1955; Lunell et al. 1982). Uterine blood flow increases slowly in early gestation and then rapidly after the second trimester, paralleling the increase in fetal mass. More precise data regarding the magnitude and timing of cardiac output, blood volume and uterine blood flow changes during pregnancy can be obtained from animal models. Fig. 2 shows data derived from Hart et al. (1985). Most of the change in stroke volume and cardiac output has already occurred by the end of the first trimester in the guinea pig, similar to the timing of these changes in human pregnancy. Interestingly, at this time there is no important change in uterine blood flow. Conversely, blood volume continues to increase at a relatively steady pace throughout pregnancy unassociated with important changes in stroke volume or cardiac output during the latter half of gestation. Thus, cardiac output and stroke volume changes appear to be temporally dissociated from uterine blood flow and blood volume increases during gestation.

4.3.2 Heart Rate

Heart rate increases are noted in all studies of human gestation but are not uniform in other mammalian species. The increase in heart rate is progressive through pregnancy (Fig. 1). Clapp (1985) measured heart rate prospectively in women planning pregnancy. His studies showed that heart rate is increased as early as 4 weeks after the last menstrual period. Heart rate change was not noted in the menstrual cycle in these women prior to pregnancy. Accordingly, these data suggest a hormonal mechanism for the increase in heart rate which is not present during the normal menstrual cycle. The mechanism for heart rate increase is unclear. Pregnant Pygmy goats showed increased rest and exercise heart rate compared to nonpregnant female controls. The difference was maintained during autonomic blockade with atropine and propranolol (Hosenpud et al. 1986). Thus, at least some of the increase in heart rate during pregnancy may be due to an increase in the intrinsic sinus node firing rate rather than alterations in autonomic control.

4.3.3 Stroke Volume

The increase in stroke volume during pregnancy was originally thought to be related to the increased blood volume and the Starling mechanism (Katz et al. 1978). Katz and others observed that left ventricular end diastolic volume assessed by echocardiography increased in concert with the increase in stroke volume during pregnancy. Ejection fraction remained unchanged or mildly increased. However, studies of left ventricular function in supine, normal subjects do not support increased venous return as a mechanism for increasing stroke volume by 30% (Parker and Case 1979). Thus, the mechanism for increased stroke volume in pregnancy clearly seemed to be that a larger end-diastolic volume ejects normally to produce a larger stroke volume. However, normal physiology suggests that we cannot have the

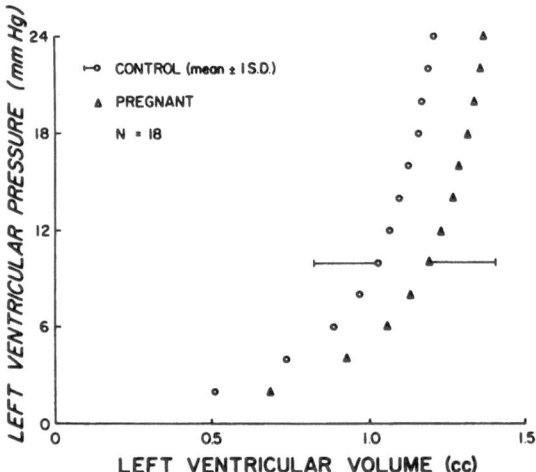

Fig. 3. Left ventricular pressure-volume curves are shown for end gestation pregnant and matched control guinea pigs. The left ventricle is larger and more compliant during guinea pig pregnancy. Hypertrophy was not present. (From Morton et al. 1984)

reported increase in end-diastolic volume from acute increases in cardiac filling pressures. Thus, the heart must remodel. In an investigation of ventricular enlargement in guinea pig pregnancy, we (Morton et al. 1984) demonstrated that the guinea pig ventricle was enlarged without hypertrophy during pregnancy (Fig. 3). This change was not associated with an alteration in material properties or the subcellular constituents. It appeared that the guinea pig ventricle was remodeled during pregnancy as a larger, thinner chamber. Subsequent investigations have shown that ventricular remodeling similar to that of pregnancy can be produced in guinea pigs (Hart et al. 1985) and in ewes (Giraud et al. 1988; Jacobson et al. 1989) by administration of estrogen. Thus, the mechanism for stroke volume increase in pregnancy appears to be cardiac enlargement through remodeling of the ventricle with normal or slightly enhanced ventricular function. It is possible that these changes are hormonally mediated.

4.3.4 Distribution of Cardiac Output

Since cardiac output is increased early in pregnancy and uterine blood flow is not, other tissues must receive increased flow. The precise distribution of this increased flow in early human pregnancy is not certain. However, kidneys (Lindheimer and Katz 1970), skin (Myhrman et al. 1980), and breasts (Pickles 1953) are recipients of increased blood flow. Since cardiac output does not change much during the second half of gestation, while uterine blood flow increases dramatically, blood flow must be distributed away from relatively plethoric areas to the enlarging uteroplacental bed. The mechanisms for early decrease in regional vascular resistance to nonuterine tissues and then the subsequent redistribution to the uterus in late gestation remain to be precisely defined.

4.4 Cardiac and Vascular Pressures

4.4.1 Systemic Arterial Pressure

Blood pressure is uniformly reduced by the second trimester of normal human pregnancy (MacGillivray 1969). Mean arterial pressure falls approximately 10 mmHg, rising to near control levels by the end of gestation. Pulse pressure is increased because of a greater fall in diastolic than in systolic pressure.

4.4.2 Venous Pressure

The venous pressure during human pregnancy is normal in the upper body (Bader et al. 1955) and increased in the lower body in supine women late in gestation (Ferris and Wilkins 1937). This latter increase occurs because of inferior vena cava compression by the pregnant uterus. The finding of normal upper extremity venous pressure despite the marked increase in blood volume suggests that either vascular capacitance or compliance, or both, are increased during pregnancy.

4.4.3 Cardiac Pressures

Right heart and pulmonary capillary wedge pressures are normal during human pregnancy and may fall in the supine posture in late gestation (Bader et al. 1955). Right atrial, right ventricular and left ventricular end diastolic pressures are not altered in guinea pig pregnancy (Morton et al. 1984; Hart et al. 1985). These findings of normal filling pressures in the heart support the concept of ventricular remodeling during pregnancy in order that a larger end diastolic volume can be accommodated at a normal filling pressure.

4.5 Vascular Resistance

Vascular resistance changes during pregnancy occur early, are striking and mirror the changes in cardiac output in humans and guinea pigs (Figs.1, 2). Since the early reduction in vascular resistance cannot be explained by the expanded uteroplacental bed, other mechanisms for vasodilation must be proposed. Generalized pressor hyporesponsiveness has been demonstrated during human and other mammalian pregnancy. These findings have been related to vasodilatory prostaglandins produced by the placenta and/or endothelium-derived relaxing factor produced locally in response to the pregnant state. The role, if any, of these factors in the vasodilatation of pregnancy remains uncertain at this time. This remains a critical area for investigation since the mechanism for the early fall in vascular resistance during pregnancy remains to be defined. In addition, understanding the mechanisms that redistribute blood to the uteroplacental circulation at the end of gestation may be important for understanding pathophysiologic processes.

4.5.1 Vascular Impedance

Vascular impedance is a quantity that describes the resistance to ejection of blood from the ventricle in a pulsatile system. In addition to vascular resistance, arterial compliance is the other major determinant of vascular impedance. Since vascular resistance is known to be markedly reduced during pregnancy, impedance is likewise reduced. This is important because this makes ventricular ejection easier. In addition, studies of the human (Hart et al. 1986) and guinea pig (Hart et al. 1989) aorta during pregnancy have shown increase in aortic size and compliance. Studies in the guinea pig also showed reduced impedance. Reduced vascular impedance during pregnancy may match the enlarged thinner left ventricle, which might otherwise find ejection more difficult without vascular remodeling. Thus, the dilated ventricle of pregnancy is nicely matched to a low impedance vascular circuit. This may allow increased stroke volume with neither changes in filling pressure nor important cardiac hypertrophy.

4.6 Vascular Capacitance

Since blood volume is markedly elevated during pregnancy and venous pressure is not, and arterial pressure is, in fact, reduced, one quickly arrives at the conclusion that the container holding the blood is larger. Mean circulatory filling pressure (MCFP), the pressure in the circulation in the absence of cardiac activity, is a measure of the fullness of the vascular compartment. Most of the vascular capacity lies in the venous system. Previous estimates of MCFP during pregnancy by Douglas et al. (1967) and Goodlin et al. (1984) revealed significant increases in MCFP during pregnancy in anesthetized dogs and rabbits. My colleagues and I (Davis et al. 1989) studied chronically instrumented guinea pigs. We were unable to detect a significant change in MCFP with pregnancy but found a marked shift to the right of the vascular mean circulatory filling pressure-volume relationship during pregnancy or estrogen administration (Fig. 4). Vascular compliance was also mildly increased during pregnancy in these studies. Thus, it appears that the vascular capacitance bed is remodeled in pregnancy, similar to the remodeling of cardiac structures and the arterial system, as a larger, more compliant structure. Vascular capacitance appears to increase at the same rate as blood volume in order that mean circulatory filling pressure is not importantly changed during pregnancy. Furthermore, estrogen may be an important mediator of this effect.

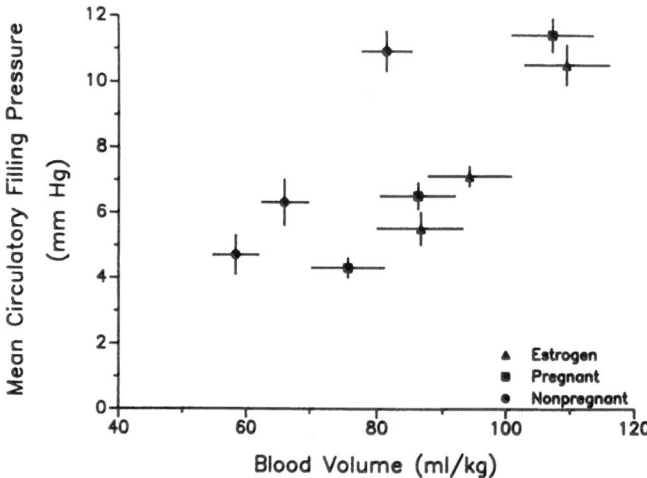

Fig. 4. Mean circulatory filling pressure (MCFP)-blood volume relationships (means ± SE) for pregnant, nonpregnant, and estrogen-treated guinea pigs. MCFP was measured during circulatory arrest at control and nominal -10% and +20% changes in blood volume. Actual blood volume changes were then calculated from blood volume measured before perturbation. Low-volume MCFP appears higher than might be expected if a single linear relationship were present, suggesting some reflex vasoconstriction during hemorrhage. Analysis of covariance demonstrates that MCFP-blood volume relationships are shifted to the right during pregnancy and estrogen administration in the guinea pig. (From Davis et al. 1989)

4.7 Summary

The cardiovascular adaptations to pregnancy are striking and may be unique, that is different from other pathophysiologic or physiologic adaptations. Sex steroids may play an important role in cardiac, arterial, and venous remodeling during pregnancy. The mechanisms for cardiovascular adaptation during pregnancy should be vigorously pursued in order to increase our understanding of this process and to develop potentially novel approaches to the treatment of cardiovascular diseases.

References

Assali NS, Rauramo L, Peltonen T (1960) Measurement of uterine blood flow and uterine metabolism: VIII. Uterine and fetal blood flow and oxygen consumption in early human pregnancy. Am J Obstet Gynecol 79:86-98

Bader RA, Bader ME, Rose DJ, Braunwald E (1955) Hemodynamics at rest and during exercise in normal pregnancy as studied by cardiac catheterization. 35:1524-1536

Clapp JF III (1985) Maternal heart rate in pregnancy. Am J Obstet Gynecol 152:659-660

Davis LE, Hohimer AR, Giraud GD, Paul MS, Morton MJ (1989) Vascular pressure-volume relationships in pregnant and estrogen-treated guinea pigs. Am J Physiol 257:R1205-R1211

Douglas BH, Harlan JC, Langford HG, Richardson TQ (1967) Effect of hypervolemia and elevated arterial pressure on circulatory dynamics of pregnant animals. Am J Obstet Gynecol 98:889-894

Ferris EB Jr, Wilkins RW (1937) The clinical value of comparative measurements of the pressure in the femoral and cubital veins. Am Heart J 13:431-439

Giraud GD, Morton MJ, Thornburg KL, Paul MS, Davis LE (1988) Estradiol produces rapid ventricular remodelling in the ewe. Society for Gynecological Investigation Program and Abstracts, 35th Annual Meeting, Baltimore p 203

Goodlin RC, Niebauer MJ, Holmberg MJ, Zucker IM (1984) Mean circulatory filling pressure in pregnant rabbits. Am J Obstet Gynecol 148:224-225

Hart MV, Hosenpud JD, Hohimer AR, Morton MJ (1985) Hemodynamics during pregnancy and sex steroid administration in guinea pigs. Am J Physiol 249:R179-R185

Hart MV, Morton MJ, Hosenpud JD, Metcalfe J (1986) Aortic function during normal human pregnancy. Am J Obstet Gynecol 154:887-891

Hart MV, Morton MJ, Gade JN (1989) Aortic remodelling during guinea pig pregnancy. Soc Gynecol Invest Scientific Abstracts, 36th Annual Meeting, San Diego, March 15-18, p 165

Hosenpud JD, Hart MV, Rowles JR, Morton MJ (1986) Maternal heart rate and stroke volume in the Pygmy goat: effects of exercise and cardiac autonomic blockade. Quart J Exp Physiol 71:59-65

Hytten FE, Paintin DB (1963) Increase in plasma volume during normal pregnancy. J Obstet Gynaecol Br Commonw 70:402-407

Jacobson S-L, Giraud GD, Morton MJ, Thornburg KL (1989) The ewe, a model for the study of cardiac adaptations during estrogen administration and hypertension. Soc Gynecol Invest Scientific Abstracts, 36th Annual Meeting, San Diego, March 15-18, p 176

Katz R, Karliner JS, Resnick R (1978) Effects of a natural volume overload state (pregnancy) on left ventricular performance in normal human subjects. Circulation 58:434-441

Kerr MG, Scott DB, Samuel E (1964) Studies of the inferior vena cava in late pregnancy. Br Med J 1:532-533

Letsky E (1980) The haematological system. In: Hytten F, Chamberlain G (Eds) Clinical physiology in obstetrics. Blackwell, Oxford

Lindheimer MD, Katz AI (1970) The kidney in pregnancy. New Engl J Med 283:1095-1097

Longo LD (1983) Maternal blood volume and cardiac output during pregnancy: a hypothesis of endocrinologic control. Am J Physiol 245:R720-R729

Lunell NO, Mylund LE, Lewander R, Sarby B (1982) Uteroplacental blood flow in pre-eclampsia measurements with indium-113m and a computer-linked gamma camera. Clin Exp Hypertension (B) 1:104-117

MacGillivray I, Rose GA, Rowe B (1969) Blood pressure survey in pregnancy. Clin Sci 37:395-407

Metcalfe J, Romney SL, Ramsey LH, Reid DE, Burwell CS (1955) Estimation of uterine blood flow in normal human pregnancy at term. J Clin Invest 34:1632-1638

Morton MJ (1990) Maternal hemodynamics in pregnancy. In: Mittelmark RA, Wiswell RA, Drinkwater BL (Eds) Exercise in pregnancy. Williams & Wilkins, Baltimore, pp 61-70

Morton M, Tsang H, Hohimer R, Ross D, Thornburg K, Faber J, Metcalfe J (1984) Left ventricular size, output and structure during guinea pig pregnancy. Am J Physiol 246:R40-R48

Myhrman P, Jansson I, Lundgren Y (1980) Skin blood flow in normal pregnancy measured by venous occlusion plethysmography of the hand. Acta Obstet Gynecol Scand 59:107-110

Parker JO, Case RB (1979) Normal left ventricular function. Circulation 60:4-11

Pickles VR (1953) Blood flow estimations as indices of mammary activity. J Obstet Gynaecol Br Emp 60:301-311

Robson SC, Hunter S, Boys RJ, Dunlop W (1989) Serial study of factors influencing changes in cardiac output during human pregnancy. Am J Physiol 256:H1060-H1065

Ueland K, Novy MJ, Peterson EN, Metcalfe J (1969) Maternal cardiovascular dynamics: IV. The influence of gestational age on the maternal cardiovascular response to posture and exercise. Am J Obstet Gynecol 104:856-864

5 Oral Contraceptives and Thrombotic Risk: A Critical Overview

Eberhard F. Mammen

5.1 Epidemiological Association

The association between oral contraceptive ingestion and thromboembolic risk is, at this time, still based on epidemiological studies. While early studies spoke of "cause and effect," it is now clear that epidemiological studies can only establish an *association* between two events, but not a direct causal relationship (MacMahon 1979).

Many studies reviewed the risk of "cardiovascular disease" in oral contraceptive users. This term encompasses a large spectrum of diseases of the heart and vessels. Most studies related, however, to "thromboembolic disease," a subgroup of cardiovascular disease. This lack of specificity in terminology has led to some confusion in the interpretation of the reported results. This review addresses *thromboembolic disease* in oral contraceptive users and the references cited are selective.

Three major thromboembolic events have been studied in women on oral contraceptives: venous thrombosis with or without pulmonary embolism, acute myocardial infarction, and cerebrovascular infarcts. Cerebrovascular infarcts can, however, be either thrombotic strokes or subarachnoidal hemorrhages.

Most of the epidemiological reports were case-control rather than cohort studies. Case-control studies do not allow the calculation of absolute risk although estimates can be made when the cases are obtained from defined populations (Thorogood and Vessey 1990).

The initial information on the effects of oral contraceptives and thromboembolic disease came from the United Kingdom in the 1970s (Inman et al. 1970; Royal College of General Practitioners 1974, 1978). Subsequently, numerous similar reports were generated in several countries which were summarized and critiqued by Realini and Goldzieher (1985). These authors conclude: "Readers must be aware of the potential sources of bias in case-control, cohort, and mortality statistics studies in order to interpret such literature appropriately."

The earlier epidemiological studies on oral contraceptive users suggested for acute myocardial infarction a relative increased risk from 2 to 4, a risk of 2 to 6 for cerebrovascular accidents, and a relative risk of 8 (3 for cohort studies) for fatal pulmonary embolism (Inman and Vessey 1968; Mann et al. 1975; Royal College of General Practitioners 1978). According to Thorogood and Vessey (1990) four conclusions could be drawn from these earlier data:

1. The absolute risk for fatal cardiovascular disease seemed to increase with patient age
2. The increased risk for myocardial infarction seemed to be exacerbated by coexisting risk factors, especially cigarette smoking
3. The risk was confined to women while taking the oral contraceptive
4. The risk seemed to be influenced little by duration of treatment

Since the beginning of the 1980s two major changes occurred relative to oral contraceptives: In the new formulations the estrogen content was markedly reduced, and women below the age of 30 used oral contraceptives more often than women over 30 years of age (Thorogood and Vessey 1990).

Since then there seems to have been a marked reduction in the incidence of acute myocardial infarction, thrombotic stroke, and venous thromboembolic disease, especially fatal pulmonary embolism (Böttiger et al. 1980; Hirvonen and Idänpää-Heikkilä 1990; Thorogood and Vessey 1990). The risk for developing acute myocardial infarction while using these newer oral contraceptive formulations varies from 1.1 to 1.3; many studies no longer find an increased risk (see Realini and Goldzieher 1985). This seems to change, however, when smoking is involved (Goldbaum et al. 1987) and with age over 35 years (Layde and Beral 1987). Also the risk for thrombotic strokes has virtually disappeared. Most observed remaining cerebrovascular events seem to be due to subarachnoidal hemorrhage (relative risk 1.4) caused by ruptured aneurysms as verified by autopsy (Hirvonen and Idänpää-Heikkilä 1990).

The relative risk for venous thromboembolic disease is very difficult to assess because so many venous thromboses or pulmonary emboli are clinically not recognized. The clinical diagnosis of deep vein thrombosis is insensitive and nonspecific (Hirsh et al. 1981) and only 1% of all venous thromboses are *clinically* recognized. Similar problems exist with the diagnosis of pulmonary embolism. Therefore, associations exist only for oral contraceptive use and *fatal* pulmonary embolism. With the newer formulations a relative risk of 1.2 or less seems to be evolve (Gerstman et al. 1990), but no data are available from large epidemiological studies (Hirvonen and Idänpää-Heikkilä 1990). Again, Realinini and Goldzieher (1985) have cautioned readers for potential sources of bias in these epidemiological reports.

Overall, the incidence of thromboembolic diseases, arterial and venous, seems to be very low in users of the new oral contraceptive formulations, unless confounding factors, especially heavy smoking and age (35) are present. The risk seems to be unrelated to the length of use and seems to disappear totally when oral contraceptives are discontinued (Stampfer et al. 1990). As pointed out by these authors, this finding suggests that oral contraceptives exert a short-term effect to explain the increased risk, especially for myocardial infarction. The effects can hardly be explained by a progression of atherosclerosis.

It thus appears that the dose of estrogen determines the incidence of thromboembolic complications associated with oral contraceptive use. Mead (1988) pointed out, however, that estrogen dose would not be the sole contributing factor and that progestogen might also play a role.

It was suggested that the estrogen effect would mostly be on coagulation while the progestogen effect would be on lipid metabolism and blood pressure.

The relationship between lipid metabolism in the development of atherosclerotic disease and its interaction with oral contraceptives, especially the progesterone component, was recently reviewed by Tikkanen (1990). While most of the data summarized originated from the older formulations, the newer low-estrogen, low-progestin preparations seem to have little effect on low-density or high-density lipoprotein cholesterol distribution in plasma (Gevers-Leuven et al. 1984). In spite of the changes noted with the older formulations, there is no convincing evidence, epidemiological or experimental, that oral contraceptives are associated with an increased risk for atherosclerosis (Hoppe 1990). From the Framingham Study, it became apparent that smoking women on oral contraceptives who developed acute myocardial infarcts or thrombotic strokes had blood clots rather than atherosclerotic narrowing of their arteries (Castelli 1986).

Hypertension, if observed in conjunction with oral contraceptives, could, of course, potentially impact the incidence of cerebrovascular bleeding which, as stated before, seems to be due largely to ruptured aneurysms.

5.2 Oral Contraceptives and Hemostasis

The epidemiological association between oral contraceptives, especially the older formulations, and thromboembolic disease has prompted numerous clinical and experimental studies to find an explanation for this phenomenon. Since thrombosis is a pathogical event brought about by activation of the hemostasis system, at an inappropriate time and in an inappropriate blood vessel, most studies were directed toward the hemostasis system.

It is today generally accepted that arterial forms of thrombosis are predominantly driven and mediated by the blood platelets which respond, in most instances, to vascular lesions. Atherosclerosis is, of course, by far the most common vascular lesion at least in the Western world. Venous thrombosis is more dependent on the coagulation system although platelets must certainly participate in this event. Venous thrombi most commonly develop in regions of decreased or disturbed blood flow, such as in the large venous sinuses in the calf, in valve cusp pockets, or in venous segments following exposure to trauma (Stamatakis et al. 1978; Hull et al. 1979). In surgical patients activation of the coagulation system or inhibition of the fibrinolytic system together with decreased blood flow possibly provide the trigger for the initial thrombus formation. The role of venous endothelial injury in this event is uncertain. While microscopic injury has been found in conjunction with elective hip and knee replacements, it has never been demonstrated in other forms of surgery. Submicroscopical or metabolic endothelial damage has been postulated (Stewart et al. 1974) but has never been proven.

Also changes in the clotting or fibrinolytic systems (hypercoagulability) can contribute to thrombosis, but these alterations primarily affect the venous pathogenesis of thrombosis and to a far lesser extent arterial thrombosis.

In reviewing the literature that has accumulated regarding oral contraceptives and thrombosis, the difference between the pathogenesis of arterial and venous thrombosis has often not been considered. Decreases in antithrombin III, for example, have been described as equally responsible for venous as well as arterial thrombosis. It is well known, however, that arterial thrombosis is extremely uncommon in patients with congenital antithrombin III deficiency (Sas 1990), and those few patients who had it were older persons.

It would thus follow, if the concept is correct, that estrogen and/or progesterone must have an effect on endothelium and/or platelets in order to explain the association with acute myocardial infarction or thrombotic strokes. They must have an effect on the coagulation system or on blood flow in order to explain the association with venous thromboembolism.

Any *systemic* effect of estrogen and/or progesterone on the hemostasis system, must also reconcile two basic questions:

1. Why would a generalized state of "hypercoagulability," arterial or venous, only yield thromboembolism in so few OC users?
2. Why would some OC users get a thrombosis within the first two cycles, occasionally even within days, while others get it after years of treatment?

In the following the reported effects of oral contraceptives on the components of the hemostasis system will be critically reviewed.

5.3 Oral Contraceptives and Vascular Lesions

It was already pointed out that there is neither epidemiological nor experimental evidence that oral contraceptives foster the development of atherosclerosis (Hoppe 1990). Atherosclerosis is rare in young persons and especially rare in young women (Juergens et al. 1960), and only 10% of 520 young persons with arteriosclerosis obliterans, for example, were women. Holmes et al. (1979) studied 31 women before the age of 45 with symptomatic peripheral vascular disease and found that all were heavy smokers, 65% had hyperlipidemia, 45% had hypertension, and only 35% had ever used oral contraceptives. Atherosclerosis can thus hardly be an explanation for the association between oral contraceptives and arterial thrombotic events. Venous thrombosis would not be affected in anyway.

In 1970 Irey et al. (1970) described endothelial proliferation with or without attached thrombi in arteries and veins of 20 women who had ingested oral contraceptives. It was speculated that these lesions were estrogen related. Subsequently, the same authors (Irey and Norris 1973; Irey et al. 1978) and others (Osterholzer et al. 1977; Basdevant et al. 1980) described these lesions as *not* specific for oral contraceptive users. These reports led Taylor (1974) to suggest ". . . there are rare individuals where vascular tissues react to endogenous or exogeneous sex steroids in an idiosyncratic fashion so as to acquire proliferative intimal lesions which gradually lead to major vessel closure." Interestingly these lesions have apparently never been described again.

Little is known at this time about the effects of estrogen and/ or progesterone on endothelial cells directly or on the regulatory mechanisms through which the endothelial cells regulate hemostasis. It has become apparent in the last decade that the endothelial cell surface plays a vital role in the local regulation of hemostasis. The unperturbed endothelial cell surface has basically *anticoagulant* properties, and receptors, such as thrombomodulin, or heparin-like molecules have been identified. As the cell becomes perturbed, this anticoagulant property seems to change to a *procoagulant* posture whereby the release of tissue factor seems to play a very important role (Müller-Berghaus 1989). Equally unknown is their effect on the various proteins of the extracellular matrix which are intimately involved in cell adhesion, such as platelets, or other aspects of hemostasis (Columbatti and Bonaldo 1991). Whether estrogen and/or progesterone have an impact on this regulatory system is presently not well researched. Even if these hormones would exert a general effect, this would not satisfactorily answer the two questions raised before.

5.4 Oral Contraceptives and Platelets

Platelet function and oral contraceptives has been studied from two points of view, the role of the prostaglandin pathway in regulating platelet-endothelial cell interaction and platelet adhesion and aggregation, predominantly in vitro.

As shown in Fig. 1, the interrelationship between platelets and endothelial cells is largely governed by the prostaglandin pathway. Platelet membranes synthesize thromboxane A_2, a powerful platelet aggregating substance and a vasoconstrictor, while endothelial cell membranes produce prostacyclin or prostaglandin I_2, a powerful anti-aggregating agent and a vasodilator (Weksler 1987). Besides primary hemostasis, this homeostatic balance, when disturbed, has also been implicated in the development of early atherosclerosis (Oates et al. 1988).

Both prostacyclin and thromboxane levels and synthesis have been studied in oral contraceptive users, in in vitro cell culture experiments, and in animals. Rather contradictory results have been described. Two studies on oral contraceptive users (old formulations) seemed to show diminished inhibition of platelet aggregation by endothelial cells (Nordøy et al. 1978) and increased thromboxane A_2 production (Schorer et al. 1978). Animal studies revealed decreased prostacyclin levels and increased platelet aggregation under estrogen treatment but no changes with combination preparations (Elam et al. 1980); others found increased prostacyclin production with combination formulations (Roncaglioni et al. 1979). In umbilical vein endothelial cultures decreased formation of prostacyclin was reported with ethinyl estradiol (David et al. 1989) and increased thromboxane formation with high

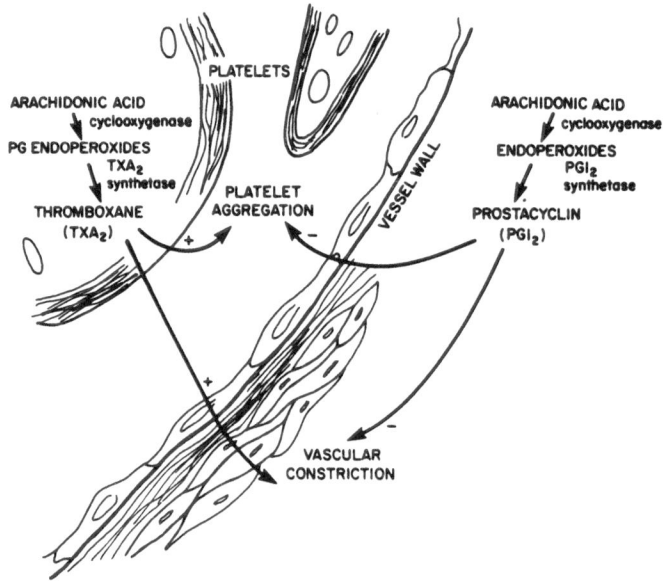

Fig. 1. Role of the prostaglandin pathway in the homeostasis between vessel wall and platelets. (From Henry 1977)

doses of the same compound (Witter and DiBlasie 1984). More recently it was shown that both estradiol alone or in combination with progesterone decreased prostacyclin production, with no significant effect on platelet aggregation or platelet thromboxane formation (Nordbø Berge et al. 1990).

The significance of these observations in the pathogenesis of arterial thrombosis in oral contraceptive users is not known at this time. Also unknown is the effect of these compounds on an alternative pathway of in vivo platelet activation, shear-induced platelet aggregation as studied by O'Brien (1990).

Changes in platelet function have also been studied in women on oral contraceptives and equally conflicting results can be found.

In part these discrepancies are due to technical problems associated with measuring platelet adhesion in particular and platelet aggregation to a lesser extent. Methods for platelet adhesion are unreliable and not standardized so that it is not surprising to find reports on increased adhesion, decreased adhesion, and no change in women taking oral contraceptive compounds (see Mammen 1982). Again most data were obtained when older formulations were widely used. Furthermore, there is little information which links increased platelet adhesion with thromboembolic disease. One report linked increased adhesion with ischemic strokes (Sharma et al. 1978).

Platelet aggregation has been studied more widely, but controversial results have been reported in users of oral contraceptives (see Mammen 1982). This again may be related to technical problems, lack of standardization and poor reproducibility of the customary aggregation techniques, using platelet-rich plasma or whole blood. Hyperaggregable platelets are usually defined as platelets that respond to less than the usual amounts of stimuli used for testing (ADP, epinephrine, collagen, thrombin, etc.). Such platelets have frequently been found in patients with arterial vascular thrombosis, but it is difficult to conclude whether the hyperaggregability contributed *to* the thrombosis or whether it is a consequence *of* the thrombosis. Familial thrombosing tendencies have been reported in conjunction with hyperaggregable platelets (O'Donnell et al. 1978) and the "sticky platelet syndrome," described by us, falls into that category (Rubenfire et al. 1986; Mammen et al. 1988). This autosomal dominant platelet abnormality presents clinically with transient ischemic attacks (TIAs) and thrombotic strokes, angina pectoris and acute myocardial infarction, and with transient or permanent occlusions of the retinal arteries. As with other congenital hypercoagulable states to be discussed later, not all affected family members have clinical symptoms. We are obviously well aware of the caution with which in vitro platelet aggregation studies have to be interpreted.

As reviewed before, oral contraceptive users were found to have increased in vitro platelet aggregation, normal aggregation, and even decreased aggregation (see Mammen 1982). Most of these data involved patients on older formulations. More recent studies in women on low-dose contraceptives, triphasic or monophasic, showed no changes in platelet aggregability (Bonnar et al. 1987; David et al. 1990; Abbate et al. 1990; Daly and Bonnar 1990). Platelet counts are unchanged in oral contraceptive users.

In the last few years so-called molecular markers of hemostasis activation have been developed which, in analogy to tumor markers, assess the presence of end products of platelet activation, thrombin or plasmin generation. This concept was reviewed by Fareed (1984). Two of these markers, platelet factor 4 and β-thromboglobulin, are end products of in vivo platelet activation and elevated plasma levels would suggest an increased in vivo platelet activation (Walz 1984). Unfortunately these markers are greatly dependent on the blood drawing and processing technique and inadequate blood handling can easily give false high plasma levels.

Few investigators have measured these two platelet release proteins either alone or in combination in oral contraceptive users. Normal levels of platelet factor 4 and β-thromboglobulin seem to be the predominant findings (Okuno and Crockat 1977; Bagdade and Subbareh 1982; Farag et al. 1988; Abbate et al. 1990; David et al. 1990). In our study we matched oral contraceptive users with corresponding female nonusers (Farag et al. 1988). While we (Farag et al. 1988) did not observe extreme values, David et al. (1990) found few women who had very high β-thromboglobulin values. This could mean that these women with high values had indeed an in vivo increased platelet activation, alternatively blood collection and handling may have been responsible for these findings. We have found that these technical problems can be greatly reduced when the blood is drawn by one or two experienced collaborators.

In general it seems, that the newer low dose oral contraceptives exert no adverse effects on platelets, especially they do not increase in vivo platelet activation, a prerequisite for the development of arterial thrombosis.

5.5 Oral Contraceptives and Coagulation

The coagulation system consists of two parts, a clotting system which leads to the formation of fibrin and a fibrinolytic system which dissolves the fibrin. There is a large body of evidence which suggests that both systems are in a continuous subliminal state of activation. This would imply that a balanced equilibrium must exist between clotting and fibrinolysis.

An imbalance between the two would obviously lead to a dysregulation, as is shown in Fig. 2. It has long been known that a defective

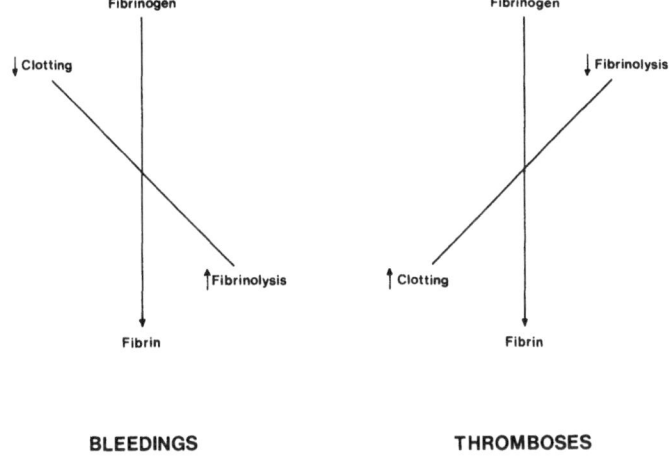

BLEEDINGS   THROMBOSES

Fig. 2. The hemostatic system as a balance between clotting and fibrinolysis. Dysregulation can lead to a hemorrhagic diathesis or to thromboembolic diseases

clotting system or an increased activation of the fibrinolytic system predisposes to hemorrhages.

Our knowledge concerning the opposite constellation, namely, an increased activation of the clotting system and a defective fibrinolytic system leading to an increased, predominantly *venous* thrombosing tendency, is relatively recent. This imbalance has been referred to as being reflective of a hypercoagulable state and several reviews have examined the factors leading to such a dysregulation (Examples: Comp 1986; Mammen and Fujii 1989).

Since oral contraceptives have been found to impact on both systems, they will be discussed separately.

5.5.1 Clotting System

The clotting system centers around the activation of prothrombin to thrombin with the subsequent conversion of fibrinogen to fibrin, as illustrated in Fig. 3. This activation is driven by several clotting factors,

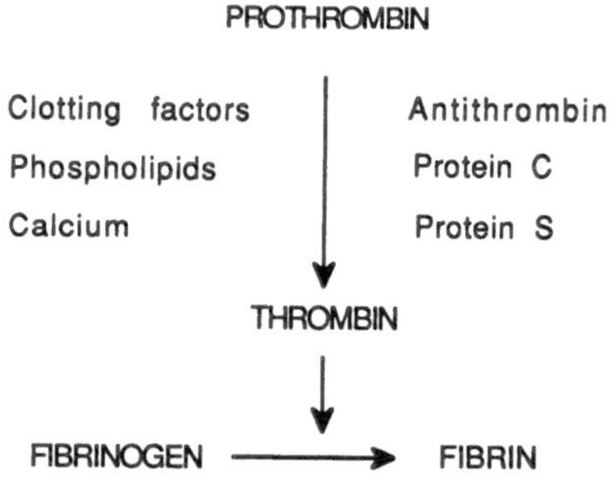

PROTHROMBIN

Clotting factors		Antithrombin
Phospholipids		Protein C
Calcium		Protein S

THROMBIN

FIBRINOGEN ⟶ FIBRIN

Fig. 3. The conversion of prothrombin to thrombin is facilitated by several clotting factors plus phospholipid surfaces and calcium. It is regulated by two inhibitor systems, antithrombin III and the protein C plus S system

some of which are proenzymes which become enzymes (prothrombin, factors X, VII, IX, XI, XII, and prekallikrein), and others are cofactors which regulate enzyme-substrate specificity (factors V, VIII, high molecular weight kininogen, and tissue factor). Some require for their proper synthesis vitamin K (prothrombin, factors X, VII, and IX). All of these interactions require negatively charged phospholipid surfaces, which are primarily derived from platelet membranes, and free calcium.

The activation is regulated by two inhibitor systems, antithrombin III and protein C plus S. Antithrombin III is a serine proteinase inhibitor. Since all clotting enzymes have a serine residue as part of their active center, all enzymes are inactivated by antithrombin III. This inactivation occurs through equimolar, irreversible complex formation. The protein C, plus S system requires the activation of protein C into its enzymic form, protein Ca. This activation is facilitated by thrombin with the aid of an endothelial cell surface bound receptor, called thrombomodulin. Protein Ca will proteolytically destroy factors V and VIII. Since factor V is the cofactor to factor Xa in the activation of prothrombin to thrombin, the elimination of this cofactor limits the *amount* of thrombin that can be generated. Factor VIII is the cofactor to factor IXa which activates factor X to factor Xa. Its destruction thus limits the *amount* of factor Xa that can be formed by this pathway.

Since this system is subliminally active at all times, the formation of thrombin must be in a state of equilibrium with its regulators. A

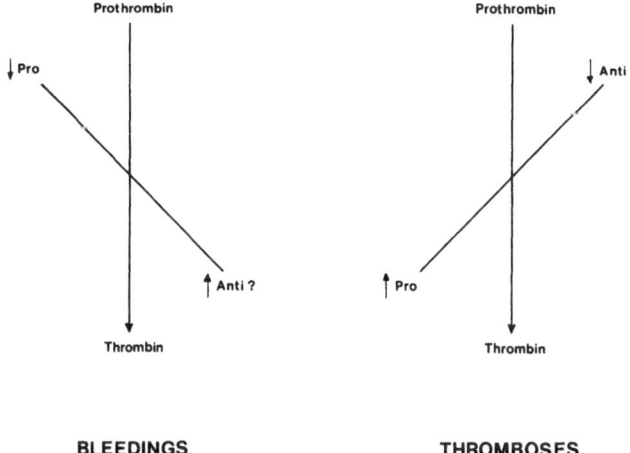

Fig. 4. An imbalance in the clotting system between procoagulants and anti-coagulants can predispose to bleedings or thromboses

dysregulation of either side of the balance could obviously lead to pathological events.

The fact that a defect in a single procoagulant factor or the presence of a pathological inhibitor can lead to bleeding, as shown in Fig. 4, has again been known for a long time (increased levels of antithrombin III, protein C or protein S are apparently not associated with a hemorrhagic tendency). That increased thrombin generation or decreased regulation of clotting can be associated with a predominantly venous thrombosis tendency has, again, only relatively recently been fully appreciated.

Most of the studies performed on the effect of oral contraceptives on the hemostasis system addressed changes in the clotting system and an enormous volume of literature has been generated. Considerable confusion was created, in part due to technical problems with the assay of the components and in part due to inappropriate data interpretation. Also the term "hypercoagulability" has been used to describe a variety of different findings, some of which, as is known now, have little to do with hypercoagulability.

Almost all studies included the two most commonly used screening tests for detecting a defect in the system, partial thromboplastin times

(APTT) and prothrombin time (PT). Both tests were originally designed to detect a deficiency of clotting factors which might lead to bleeding. Although the tests are generally reliable (within limits) for this purpose, they do respond to a variety of changes in factor levels, especially fibrinogen.

Most patients on oral contraceptives have shortened APTTs and PTs, more so with the older formulations than with the new ones. In the older literature this has been interpreted as a sign of "hypercoagulability" (see Mammen 1982). Very likely this is due to the elevated fibrinogen levels which are seen in most oral contraceptive users. There is no clinical or experimental evidence that shortened APTT and PT are signaling a prethrombotic state. Most patients with *ongoing* thrombosis have normal values and when APTTs are short, one invariably finds markedly elevated factor VIII:C and fibrinogen levels. Both proteins are acute phase reactants.

Except for the request by governmental regulatory agencies, there is no scientific merit in performing PTs and APTTs (*prolonged* APTTs may be helpful in the diagnosis of factor XII and prekallikrein deficiencies which *may* predispose to thrombosis).

The next question that needs discussion relates to elevated clotting factor levels and their relationship to thrombosis. Clotting factor levels have been extensively studied in users of oral contraceptives, and generally, increased levels have been found. With the older higher estrogen formulations virtually all factors were found to be increased. With the newer compounds fibrinogen and some of the vitamin K-dependent factors may still be affected (Omsjø et al. 1989; David et al. 1990). Others have not found significant alterations in fibrinogen levels (Notelovitz et al. 1987; Farag et al. 1988). We have recently completed a study on a new triphasic oral contraceptive and the changes noted in fibrinogen are illustrated in Fig. 5. Although the fibrinogen levels were significantly ($p < 0.001$) elevated over 12 cycles, only few patients had values outside of the normal range. The interest in fibrinogen levels in this context comes from recently conducted prospective epidemiological studies in which a positive correlation was found between plasma fibrinogen levels, plasma factor VII levels, and subsequent cardiovascular events such as acute myocardial infarction, sudden death, and cerebrovascular accidents. These studies were recently extensively summarized by Hultin (1991). For fibrinogen this associ-

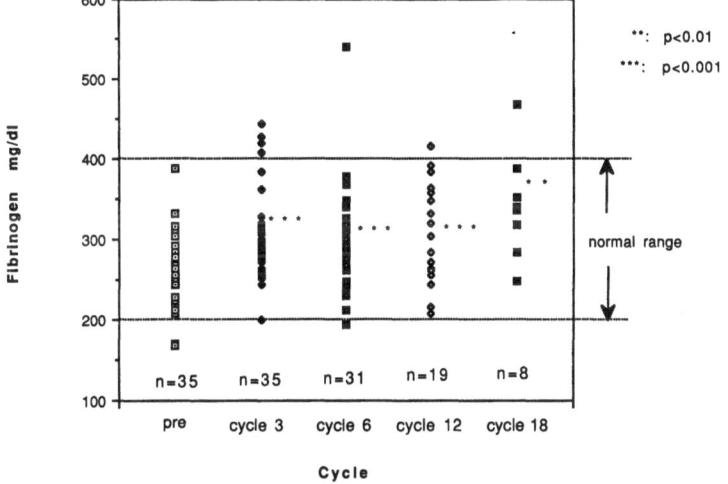

Fig. 5. Fibrinogen levels over 18 cycles of treatment with a triphasic oral contraceptive

ation was found in both men and women (two studies); for factor VII the association was found only in men. In the studies cited, the association was with extensive atherosclerosis and suggestions were made that excessive fibrinogen levels might foster platelet aggregation and an incorporation of fibrin into atheromatous plaques (Lowe 1986). Increased plasma fibrinogen levels could also increase blood viscosity (Letcher et al. 1981). As pointed out before, users of oral contraceptives have neither an increased risk for atherosclerosis nor do they have increased platelet aggregability. Attempting to use these data to explain the association between oral contraceptives and thrombosis, especially arterial, as has been done by Kelleher (1990) is speculative and lacks at this time a clinical or experimental basis. It must also be kept in mind that fibrinogen is an acute phase reactant protein so that elevations are seen with a variety of other disease states.

Changes in other coagulation factors have also been studied extensively by numerous investigators and increases have been noted with practically all procoagulants. This seems to be a general effect of estrogen on protein synthesis, and with older formulation greater in-

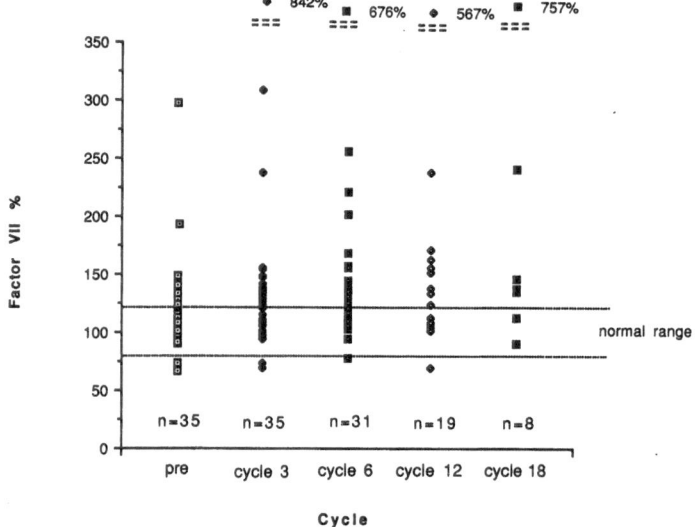

Fig. 6. Factor VII levels over 18 cycles of treatment with a triphasic oral contraceptive

creases were seen. But even low-dose estrogen formulations still exert increased synthesis. In our recent study we found clearly elevated levels of factor X, factor VII, factor VIII:C, and von Willebrand factor antigen. Factor V levels were unchanged. In the case of factor X many women had values above the upper normal range, which was less the case for factor VIII:C and von Willebrand factor. Most of those changes were increases within the established normal range for our laboratory. Factor VII showed a very unusual pattern with already many high values before treatment. During treatment two patients had consistently extremely high levels, as can be seen from Fig. 6. This cannot be due to technical assay inconsistencies.

While there is, again, no experimental evidence that higher factor levels in plasma are causing hypercoagulability for reasons outlined before (Mammen, 1982), factor VII, like fibrinogen, was associated with increased cardiovascular events (Hultin 1991). Factor VII requires tissue factor which could be liberated from atherosclerotic plaques (Kelleher 1990). Oral contraceptive users have no increased risk for atherosclerosis, as outlined above, so that the link between factor VII levels and arterial thromboembolism in oral contraceptive users (Kelleher 1990; Meade 1988) remains speculative.

The only convincing clinical evidence that the infusion of certain factors causes thrombosis comes from hemophilia B patients treated with so-called factor IX concentrates. It is well recoginized that some of these concentrates contain active enzymes, factors VIIa, Xa and IXa. An infusion of enzymes could obviously trigger clotting. The newly synthesized factors (estrogen effect) are proenzymes, however.

Therefore, there is at present little evidence which suggests that increased factor levels in plasma shift the equilibrium between pro- and anticoagulants into a hypercoagulable posture.

Decreases in antithrombin III, protein C, and protein S, on the other hand, can be associated with an increased thrombosing tendency. This is well known for patients with congenital defects of these three proteins (Comp 1986; Mammen and Fujii 1989).

Congenital antithrombin III deficiency was first described in 1965 (Egeberg 1965). Since then several other families have been observed. The vast majority of patients are heterozygotes with plasma levels between 20% and 60%. Also numerous acquired antithrombin III deficiencies have been found, and the general consensus seems to be that plasma levels under 60% place a patient at risk. The clinical manifestations are predominantly venous thrombosis.

In early 1970, von Kaulla et al. (1971) reported decreased antithrombin III levels in women taking oral contraceptives. These authors assayed antithrombin III in serum rather than plasma. This test is heavily influenced by the level of prothrombin in plasma, and when these levels are increased, as in oral contraceptive user, more thrombin is generated during the test procedure in vitro leading to greater consumption of antithrombin. Therefore, these early reports must now be considered as erroneous. Many other investigators used the same technique (see Mammen 1982). Even when antithrombin III was assayed in plasma, discrepant results were reported. In earlier studies this was probably due to the lack of standardization of the employed techniques. Even if one were to ignore these considerations, antithrombin III levels rarely were found to be under 60%.

Since the introduction of the lower estrogen containing oral contraceptives very few, if any, changes were described in antithrombin III

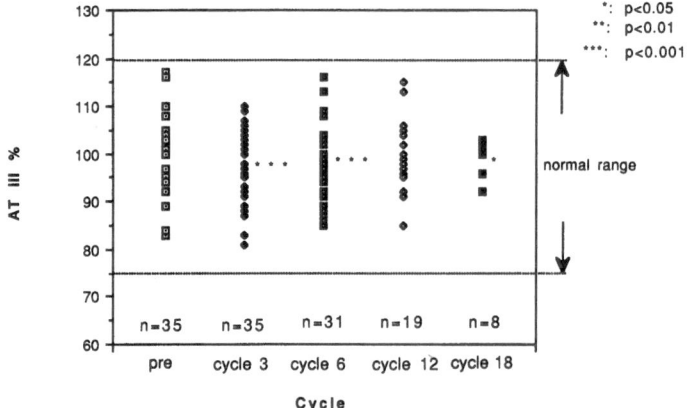

Fig. 7. Antithrombin III activity levels over 18 cycles of treatment with a triphasic oral contraceptives

levels (Bonnar et al. 1987; Notelovitz et al. 1987; Farag et al. 1988; Omsjø et al. 1989; Agoestina et al. 1989; Daly and Bonnar 1990; Abbate et al. 1990; David et al. 1990; Jespersen et al. 1990). Our recent results with a new triphasic oral contraceptive is illustrated in Fig. 7. While the decrease in antithrombin III is statistically highly significant ($p < 0.001$) during cycles 3 and 6, the change is obviously *clinically* irrelevant. The newer assays are very precise and reproducible. For example, our pretreatment mean values were 101.4% ± 8.06, the values at cycle 3 were 96.6% ± 7.03 ($p < 0.001$). It should be apparent that decreases in antithrombin III during treatment with oral contraceptives cannot explain the increased risk of thrombosis. Moreover it would only apply to venous thromboembolism.

There are fewer reports on protein C in women taking oral contraceptives and all involve the newer formulations. While we observed a significant increase in plasma protein C levels (Farag et al. 1988), others found no changes (Gilabert et al. 1988; Jespersen et al. 1990; Abbate et al. 1990). Patients with congenital protein C deficiency are overwhelmingly heterozygotes with plasma levels under 50%, and considerable variability has been found in the general population (Miletich et al. 1987). Most clinical manifestations are venous thromboembolism, but occasionally a patient with arterial thrombosis at unusual sites is noted. Since oral contraceptives do not alter or even increase protein C levels, the high risk for thrombosis cannot be explained on that basis either.

The cofactor to protein C, protein S, has so far only scarcely been studied in oral contraceptive users (Boerger et al. 1987; Gilabert et al. 1988). Users had an 18% decrease in their protein S antigen levels (Boerger et al. 1987). This is by itself not enough to bring levels to those of heterozygous congenital protein S deficiency patients (Engesser et al. 1987) but more research is needed to fully understand this particular finding. Future studies should encompass functional protein S assays which were not readily available until recently. Also assays of levels of C4b-binding protein should be included since functional protein S levels are greatly influenced by changing levels of this component of the complement system. C4b-binding protein is an acute phase reactant protein.

A second antithrombin which circulates in plasma is heparin-cofactor II. Decreases have been found in patients with thrombosis. One study revealed significantly elevated levels of this protein in oral contraceptive users (Massouh et al. 1989).

5.5.2 Fibrinolytic System

The fibrinolytic system can be considered as another balance in which plasminogen is converted to plasmin. This conversion is driven by profibrinolytic forces and regulated by antifibrinolytic proteins. As can be seen from Fig. 8, an imbalance can predispose to bleeding, but also to thrombosis.

The main activator of plasminogen seems to be tissue plasminogen activator (t-PA). This enzyme is released from endothelial cells in response to various stimuli. t-PA is inhibited by a special regulator, called plasminogen activator inhibitor (PAI). Since so far three different inhibitors have been found, the main physiological one is referred to as PAI-1. Plasmin itself is inhibited by α_2-antiplasmin.

In the last decade evidence has been accumulating that decreases in plasminogen, decreases in t-PA release, and elevated levels of PAI-1 can predispose to thromboembolic disease (Lijnen and Collen 1989).

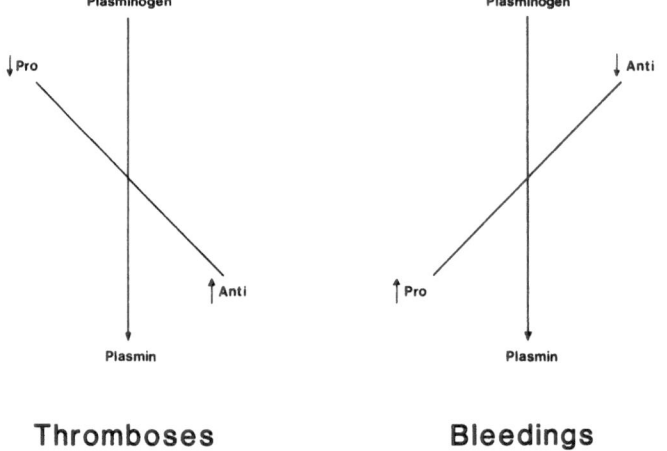

Thromboses   **Bleedings**

Fig. 8. An imbalance in the fibrinolytic system between profibrinolytic and antifibrinolytic forces can predispose to bleeding or thrombosis

Some of these fibrinolytic components have also been determined in oral contraceptive users and most information was obtained with the newer formulations.

The frequently employed screening test for fibrinolysis is whole blood or plasma euglobulin lysis times. While this is not an accurate test, shorter times, i.e., increased fibrinolysis, seems to be the predominant finding in oral contraceptive users (Bonnar et al. 1987; Agoestina et al. 1989; Abbate et al. 1990; Jespersen et al. 1990; David et al. 1990; Daly and Bonnar 1990). This would suggest that the overall fibrinolytic activity in oral contraceptive users is increased. It has been pointed out that the increased clotting, interpreted by some, would be balanced by the increased fibrinolysis, thus counteracting a potential imbalance (Gram et al. 1990; Bonnar et al. 1987).

Plasminogen levels were uniformly found to be elevated in oral contraceptive users (Bonnar et al. 1987; Farag et al. 1988; Notelovitz et al. 1987; Abbate et al. 1990; Jespersen et al. 1990; David et al. 1990; Daly and Bonnar 1990). Thrombosis is seen in patients with marked *decreases* in plasminogen levels so that the observed changes cannot link thrombosis with oral contraceptive use.

The balance between t-PA and PAI-1 has been studied less frequently in oral contraceptive users. Increased t-PA levels and decreased PAI-1 levels have been noted (Jespersen et al. 1990; Gram et al. 1990) although these results may have been influenced by technical considerations (Kooistra et al. 1990), and t-PA levels may actually be decreased. It is thus unclear at this time whether a diminished fibrinolytic potential in oral contraceptive users represents a link between thrombosis and oral contraceptive use. For the moment it seems that fibrinolysis may be increased.

Thrombosing tendency is usually associated with decreased t-PA release and elevated levels of PAI-1. α_2-Antiplasmin levels seem to remain in normal range when oral contraceptives are used (Notelovitz et al. 1987; Farag et al. 1988).

All of these at times discrepant observations made on clotting and fibrinolysis in oral contraceptive users raise the important question of whether these tests are really suited to determine a state of hypercoagulability. After all, thrombosis is a local process that may not necessarily find a reflection in an alteration of the systemic balance of factors of clotting and fibrinolysis. It is well known that most coagulation tests are normal in patients with a clinically apparent and ongoing thrombotic process. This problem has been recently critically examined by Kluft (1990).

The traditional tests to study clotting and fibrinolysis seem not to be suited to unequivocally determine a true state of hypercoagulability with accuracy. They can undoubtedly indicate a potential predisposition to thromboembolic complications, but they cannot establish the presence of this clinical problem.

This dilemma has led, in recent years, to the development of a different technology that addresses the presence of markers of thrombin or plasmin, the key enzymes of the clotting and fibrinolytic system. This technology was already briefly mentioned when platelet activation in vivo was addressed. While many different markers of hemostasis activation are being developed, four have so far found fairly wide use. These are thrombin/antithrombin III (TAT) complexes, fibrinopeptide A, prothrombin fragment 1+2, and D-dimer.

TAT complex determination makes use of a monoclonal antibody which recognizes only complexes formed between thrombin and its main inhibitor antithrombin III. There is no cross-reactivity with the individual parts that comprise the complex (Pelzer et al. 1988). In order to have TAT complexes, thrombin must have been present, i.e., the clotting system must have been activated at the time the sample was drawn. TAT complexes are stable and have a long half-life in blood.

Fibrinopeptide A is another marker of thrombin because this peptide is cleaved from fibrinogen by thrombin (Nossel et al. 1975). It was recently found that plasmin and t-PA might also release fibrinopeptide A. This limits somewhat the specificity of this assay. The peptide also has a very short half-life and is technically more difficult to assay than TAT complexes.

Prothrombin fragment 1+2 is generated from prothrombin when factor Xa cleaves the molecule (Bauer et al. 1988; Pelzer et al. 1989). It is thus another marker of clotting although not thrombin directly.

D-Dimers are split products of fibrin, not fibrinogen, and are generated when plasmin destroys fibrin. Since the formation of fibrin requires thrombin, D-dimer is a marker for the presence of both, thrombin and plasmin.

While this new technology is not yet widely available, only limited information can be found, especially as it relates to oral contraceptives. One major problem which makes these tests difficult to interpret is the effect that a poor blood draw or an improper blood handling can have on these results. Abnormal values must therefore be repeated on a newly drawn sample. We have limited this problem by having blood drawn and processed by only two experienced persons.

In one study (Abbate et al. 1990) elevated fibrinopeptide A levels were found with a monophasic and triphasic oral contraceptive. This was interpreted as evidence for an activation of the clotting system by oral contraceptives. While the authors do not state the normal range for fibrinopeptide A in their laboratory, the changes noted are well within normal range of most laboratories. We have not seen elevated fibrinopeptide A levels in oral contraceptive users (Farag et al. 1988), especially not when comparisons were made with matched controls.

TAT complexes were found to be elevated ($p < 0.01$) in oral contraceptive users by Gram et al. (1990). Looking at the scatterogram provided, about one third of the control group had levels well above the stated normal range as did about one third of the oral contraceptive users. Based on our experience, these data suggest problems with

Table 1. TAT complexes and prothrombin fragment 1+2 in women on a variety of different oral contraceptives

	TAT complexes	Fragment 1+2
Normal range	1 – 5 ng/l	0.36 – 0.95 nM/l
Oral contraceptive users	1.9 ± 0.5	0.82 ± 0.42
(n = 56)		
Controls (n = 47)	2.5 ± 1.0	0.79 ± 0.3

Mean ± SD

blood procurement and handling. The same group of investigators (Jespersen et al. 1990) found less of a change when they compared two formulations of oral contraceptives.

We have recently analyzed TAT complexes and prothrombin fragment 1+2 in 56 women taking a variety of low dose and sequential oral contraceptives and 47 controls (Saleh et al. 1991). The data listed in Table 1 suggest that there was no in vivo activation of the clotting system in these women.

It thus appears that there is no evidence for an activated clotting system in vivo in women on oral contraceptives. We are, therefore, at this time unable to explain the epidemiological association between oral contraceptive use and thromboembolic disease, as low as this association may be with the newer formulations.

The only plausible explanation could be that those women who develop thromboembolic complications while on oral contraceptives could have an unrecognized, preexisting defect in their hemostatic system. In one of our studies (Farag et al. 1988) we observed one woman with low antithrombin III levels (69%) and a positive family history for thrombosis. Canonical correlation analysis yielded a negative correlation between antithrombin levels and history of thrombosis ($r = -0.28$).

These findings, as limited as they are, probably support the manufacturers' recommendations that women with a positive personal or family history for thromboembolic disease should seek alternative contraceptive devices.

References

Abbate R, Pintos S, Rostagno C, Bruni U, Rosati D, Mariani G (1990) Effects of long-term gestodene-containing oral contraceptive administration on hemostasis. Am J Obst Gynecol 163:424-430

Agoestina T, Sabarudin U, Hoppe G (1989) A study comparing a gestogen triphasic formulation with a fixed combination OC. Adv Contraception 5:71-84

Bagdade JD, Subbareh PV (1982) Atherosclerosis and oral contraceptive use. Arteriosclerosis 2:170-176

Basdevant A, de Lignieres B, Mauais-Jarvis P (1980) Effets des contraceptifs oraux sur la paroi des vaisseaux. Nouvelle Présse Médicale 16:519-523

Bauer KA, Broekmans AW, Bertina RM, Conard J, Horellou M-H, Samama MM, Rosenberg RD (1988) Hemostatic enzyme generation in the blood of patients with hereditary protein C deficiency. Blood 71:1418-1426

Boerger LM, Morris PC, Thurnau GR, Esmon CT, Comp PC (1987) Oral contraceptives and gender affect protein S status. Blood 69:692-694

Bonnar J, Daly L, Carroll E (1987) Blood coagulation with a combination pill containing gestadene and ethinyl estradiol. Int J Fert Supplement, 21-28

Boettiger LE, Boman G, Eklund G, Westerholm B (1980) Oral contraceptives and thromboembolic disease: Effects at lowering oestrogen content. Lancet 1:1098-1101

Castelli WP (1986) The triglyceride issue: A view from Framingham. Am Heart J 112:432-437

Columbatti A, Bonaldo P (1991) The superfamily of proteins with von Willebrand factor type A-like domains: One theme common to components of extracellular matrix, hemostasis, cellular adhesion, and defense mechanisms. Blood 77:2305-2315

Comp PC (1986) Hereditary disorders predisposing to thrombosis. Progr Hemost Thromb 8:71-102

Daly L, Bonnar J (1990) Comparative studies of 30 g ethinyl estradiol combined with gestodene and desogestrel on blood coagulation, fibrinolysis, and platelets. American Journal of Obstetrics and Gynecology 163:430-437

David JL, Gaspard UJ, Gillain D, Raskinet R, Lepot MR (1990) Hemostasis profile in women taking low-dose oral contraceptives. Am J Obst Gynecol 163:420-423

David M, Griesmacher A, Müller MM (1989) 17α-Ethinyl-estradiol decreases production and release of prostacyclin in cultured human umbilical vein endothelial cells. Prostaglandins 38:431-439

Egeberg O (1965) Inherited antithrombin III deficiency causing thrombophilia. Thromb Diath Haemorrh 13:516-530

Elam MB, Lipscomb GE, Chesney CM, Terragno DA, Terragno NA (1980) Effect of synthetic estrogen on platelet aggregation and vascular release of PGI$_2$-like material in the rabbit. Prostaglandins 20:1039-1049

Engesser L, Broeckmans AW, Briet E, Brommer EJ, Bertina RM (1987) Hereditary protein S deficiency: Clinical manifestations. Ann Intern Med 106:677-682

Farag AM, Bottoms SF, Mammen EF, Hosni MA, Ali AA, Moghissi KS (1988) Oral contraceptives and the hemostasis system. Obstet Gynecol 71:584-588

Fareed J, Guest Editor (1984) Molecular markers of hemostatic disorders. Semin Thromb Hemost 10:215-332

Gerstman BB, Piper JM, Freiman JP, Tomita DK, Kennedy DL, Ferguson WJ, Bennett RC (1990) Oral contraceptive oestrogen and progestin potencies and the incidence of deep venous thromboembolism. Int J Epidemiol 19:931-936

Gevers-Leuven JA, Havekes L, vander Kooij-Poutier HA, Starmans RJH, Jansen H, Bouwhuis-Hoogerwerf ML, de Pagter HATh, Hessel LW (1984) Effect of low-dose oral contraceptives on lipoproteins and lipolytic enzymes: Differences between two commonly used preparations. Metabolism 33:1039-1042

Gilabert J, Fernandez JA, Espana F, Aznar J, Estelles A (1988) Physiological coagulation inhibitors (protein S, protein C and antithrombin III) in severe preeclamptic states and in uses of oral contraceptives. Thromb Res 49:319-329

Goldbaum GM, Kendrick JS, Hogelin GC, Gentry EM (1987) The relative impact of smoking and oral contraceptive use in women in the United States. J Am Med Ass 258:1339-1342

Gram J, Munkvad S, Jespersen J (1990) Enhanced generation and resolution of fibrin in women above the age of 30 years using oral contraceptives low in estrogen. Am J Obst Gynecol 163:438-442

Henry RL (1977) Semin Thromb Hemost 4:93-122

Hirsh J, Genton E, Hull R (1981) Venous thromboembolism. Grune and Stratton, New York, pp 73-81

Hirvonen E, Idänpään-Heikkilä J (1990) Cardiovascular death among women under 40 years of age using low-estrogen oral contraceptives and intrauterine devices in Finland from 1975 to 1984. Am J Obst Gynecol 163:281-284

Holmes DR Jr, Burbank MK, Fulton RE, Bernatz PE (1979) Arteriosclerosis obliterans in young women. Am J Med 66:997-1000

Hoppe G (1990) The clinical relevance of oral contraceptive pill-induced plasma lipid changes: Facts or fiction. Am J Obst Gynecol 163:388-391

Hull R, Hirsh J, Sackett DL, Powers P, Turpie AGG, Walker I, McBride J (1979) The value of adding impedance plethysmography to ^{125}I-fibrinogen leg scanning for the detection of deep-vein thrombosis in high-risk surgical patients: A comparative study between patients undergoing general surgery and hip surgery. Thromb Res 15:227-234

Hultin MB (1991) Fibrinogen and factor VII as risk factors in vascular disease. Progr Hemost Thromb 10:215-241

Inman WHW, Vessey MP (1968) Investigation of deaths from pulmonary, coronary and cerebral thrombosis and embolism in women of childbearing
age. Br Med J 2:193-199

Inman WHW, Vessey MP, Westerholm B, Engelund A (1970) Thromboembolic disease and the steroidal content of oral contraceptives: A report to
the Committee on Safety of Drugs. Br Med J 2:203-209

Irey NS, Norris HJ (1973) Intimal vascular lesions associated with female reproductive steroids. Arch of Path 96:227-234

Irey NS, Manion WC, Taylor HB (1970) Vascular lesions in women taking
oral contraceptives. Arch of Path 89:1-8

Irey NS, McAllister HA, Henry JM (1978) Oral contraceptives and stroke
in young women: A clinicopathologic correlation. Neurology 28:1216-
1219

Jespersen J, Petersen KR, Skouby SO (1990) Effects of new oral contraceptives on the inhibition of coagulation and fibrinolysis in relation to dosage
and type of steroid. Am J Obst Gynecol 163:396-403

Juergens JL, Barker NW, Hines EA Jr (1960) Arteriosclerosis obliterans: Review of 520 cases with special reference to pathogenic and prognostic factors. Circulation 21:188-195

Kelleher CC (1990) Clinical aspects of the relationship between oral contraceptives and abnormalities of the hemostatic system: Relation to the development of cardiovascular disease. Am J Obst Gynecol 163:392-395

Kluft C (1990) Disorders of the hemostatic system and the risk of the development of thrombotic and cardiovascular diseases: Limitations of laboratory diagnosis. Am J Obst Gynecol 163:305-312

Kooistra T, Bosma PJ, Jespersen J, Kluft C (1990) Studies on the mechanism
of action of oral contraceptives with regard to fibrinolytic variables. Am J
Obst Gynecol 163:404-412

Layde PM, Beral V (1987) Further analysis of mortality in oral contraceptive
users: Royal College of General Practioners' Oral Contraceptive Study.
Lancet 1:541-546

Letcher RL, Chien S, Pickering TG, Sealey JE, Laragh JH (1981) Direct relationship between blood pressure and blood viscosity in normal and hypertensive subjects. Role of fibrinogen and concentration. Am J Med 70:1195-
1202

Lijnen HR, Collen D (1989) Congenital and acquired deficiencies of components of the fibrinolytic system and their relation to bleeding and thrombosis. Fibrinolysis 3:67-77

Lowe GDO (1986) Blood rheology in arterial disease. Clin Sci 71:137-146

MacMahon B (1979) Strength and limitations of epidemiology, The National
Research Council in 1979: Current issues and studies. Washington, DC,
National Academy of Sciences

Mammen EF (1982) Oral contraceptives and blood coagulation: A critical review. Am J Obst Gynecol 142:781-790

Mammen EF, Fujii Y (1989) Hypercoagulable states. Lab Med 20:611-616

Mammen EF, Barnhart MI, Selik NR, Gilroy J, Klepach GL (1988) Sticky platelet syndrome: A congenital platelet abnormality predisposing to thrombosis? Folia Haematol (Leipzig) 115:340-345

Mann JI, Thorogood M, Waters WE, Powell C (1975) Oral contraceptives and myocardial infarction in young women: A further report. Br Med J 3:631-632

Massouh M, Jatoi A, Gordon EM, Ratnoff OD (1989) Heparin cofactor II activity in plasma during pregnancy and oral contraceptive use. J Lab Clin Med 114:697-699

Meade TW (1988) Risks and mechanisms of cardiovascular events in users of oral contraceptives. Am J Obst Gynecol 158:1646-1652

Miletich J, Sherman L, Broze G Jr (1987) Absence of thrombosis in subjects with heterozygous protein C defiency. N Engl J Med 317:991-995

Mueller-Berghaus G (1989) Pathophysiology and biochemical events in disseminated intravascular coagulation: Dysregulation of procoagulant and anticoagulant pathways. Semin Thromb Hemost 15:58-87

Norbhø Berge L, Hansen J-B, Svensson B, Lyngmo V, Nordoy A (1990) Female sex hormones and platelet endothelial cell interactions. Haemostasis 20:313-320

Nordøy A, Svensson B, Haycraft D, Hoak JC, Wiebe D (1978) The influence of age, sex, and the use of oral contraceptives on the inhibitory effects of endothelial cells and PGI_2 (prostacyclin) on platelet function. Scandinavian Journal of Haematology 21:177-187

Nossel HL, Butler VP Jr, Canfield RE, Yudelman I, Ti M, Spanondis K, Soland T (1975) Potential use of fibrinopeptide A measurements in the diagnosis and management of thrombosis. Thrombosis et Diathesis Haemorrhagica 33:426-434

Notelovitz M, Zauner C, McKenzie L, Suggs Y, Fields C, Kitchens C (1987) The effect of low-dose oral contraceptives on cardiorespiratory function, coagulation, and lipids in exercising young women: A preliminary report. Am J Obst Gynecol 156:591-598

Oates JA, FitzGerald GA, Branch RA, Jackson EK, Knapp HR, Roberts LR (1988) Clinical implications of prostaglandin and thromboxane formation. N Engl J Med 319:689-698

O'Brien JR (1990) Shear-induced platelet aggregation. Lancet 335:711-713

O'Donnell FN Jr, Carvalho ACA, Colman RW, Clowes GHA (1978) Platelet function abnormalities in a family with recurrent arterial thrombosis. Surgery 83:144-150

Okuno T, Crockat E (1977) Platelet factor 4 activity and thromboembolic episodes. Am J Clin Pathol 67:351-355

Omsjø IH, Øian P, Maltau JM, Østerud B (1989) Effects of two triphasic oral contraceptives containing ethinylestradiol plus levonorgestrel or gestodene on blood coagulation and fibrinolysis. Acta Obstet Gynecol Scand Suppl 68:27-30

Osterholzer HO, Grillo D, Kruger PS, Dunnihoo DR (1977) The effect of oral contraceptive steroids on branches of the uterine artery. Obstet Gynecol 49:227-232

Pelzer H, Schwarz H, Heimburger N (1988) Determination of human throm-
bin/antithrombin III complex in plasma with an enzyme-linked immunosorbent assay. Thrombosis and Haemostasis 59:101-106

Pelzer H, Stüber W (1989) Markers of hemostatic activation: New perspective-
s using immunochemical methods for determination of prothrombin fragment 1+2 and thrombin-antithrombin III complex. Thromb Haemost
62:165 (Abstract)

Realini JP, Goldzieher JW (1985) Oral contraceptives and cardiovascular disease:
A critique of the epidemiologic studies. Am J Obst Gynecol 152:729-798

Roncoglioni MC, DiMinno G, Regers I, de Gaetano G, Donati MB (1979) Increased prostacyclin-like activity in vascular tissues from rats on long-term treatment with an oestrogen-progestogen combination. Thromb Res 14:793-797

Royal College of General Practitioners (1974) Oral contraceptives and health.
Pitman, London

Royal College of General Practitioners (1978) Oral contraceptives, venous
thrombosis, and varicose veins. Journal of the Royal College of General
Practioners 28:393-399

Rubenfire M, Blevins RD, Barnhart M, Householder S, Selik N, Mammen EF
(1986) Platelet hyperaggregability in patients with chest pain and angio-
graphically normal coronary arteries. Am J Cardiol 57:657-660

Saleh AA, Brockbank N, Dorey LG, Ozawa T, Dombrowski MP, Bottoms SF,
Cotton DB, Mammen EF (1992) Molecular markers of hemostasis activation in oral contraceptive users. Thromb Res (in print)

Sas G (1990) Clinical significance and laboratory diagnosis of antithrombin III
deficiencies. In: Sas G (Ed) The Biology of Antithrombins. CRC Press,
Boca Raton pp 33-88

Schorer AE, Gerard JM, White JG, Krivit W (1978) Oral contraceptive use alters the balance of platelet prostaglandin and thromboxane synthesis. Prostaglandins and Medicine 1:5-11

Sharma SC, Vijayan GP, Seth HN, Suri ML (1978) Platelet adhesiveness,
plasma fibrinogen, and fibrinolytic activity in young patients with ischaemic stroke. J Neurol Neurosurg Psychiatry 41:118-121

Stamatakis JD, Kakkar UV, Lawrence D, Bentley PG (1978) The origin of
thrombi in the deep veins of the lower limb: A venographic study. Br J
Surg 65:449-451

Stampfer MJ, Willett WC, Colditz GA, Speizer FE, Hennekens CH (1990) Past
use of oral contraceptives and cardiovascular disease: A meta-analysis in the
context of the Nurses' Health Study. Am J Obst Gynecol 163:285-291

Stewart GJ, Ritchie WGM, Lynch PR (1974) Venous endothelial damage produced by massive sticking and emigration of leukocytes. Am J Pathol
74:507-532

Taylor ES (1974) Editorial comment. Obstet Gynecol Surv 29:182

Thorogood M, Vessey MP (1990) An epidemiological survey of cardiovascular disease in women taking oral contraceptives. Am J Obst Gynecol
163:274-281

Tikkanen MJ (1990) Role of plasma lipoproteins in the pathogenesis of atherosclerotic disease, with special reference to sex hormone effects. Am J Obst Gynecol 163:296-304

von Kaulla E, Droegemueller W, Aoki N, von Kaulla KN (1971) Antithrombin III depression and thrombin generation acceleration in women taking oral contraceptives. Am J Obst Gynecol 109:868-873

Walz DA (1984) Platelet-released proteins as molecular markers for the activation process. Semin Thromb Hemost 10:270-279

Weksler BB (1987) Platelet interactions with the blood vessel wall. In: Colman RW, Hirsh J, Marder VJ, Salzman EW (Eds) Hemostasis and Thrombosis. Basic Principles and Clinical Practice. Lippincott, Philadelphia, PA, pp 804-815

Witter FR, DiBlasi MC (1984) Effect of steroid hormones on arachidonic acid metabolites of endothelial cells. Obstet Gynecol 63:747-751

6 Studies on the Mechanisms of Action of Steroids on Coagulation and Fibrinolysis

Cees Kluft, Jan A. Gevers Leuven, and Frans M. Helmerhorst

6.1 Introduction

Sex steroids can influence the metabolism of coagulation and fibrino-lysis variables and change their plasma concentration. These effects have been documented with various formulations of oral contraceptives (OCs) and variations in effect of different formulations have been observed (Task Force on Oral Contraceptives 1991).

One obvious reason for performing studies on these changes relates to the increased risk of thromboembolic disease observed in women using OCs with a high oestrogen-type component. This paper considers

the extent to which laboratory analysis of the isolated variables of haemostasis during contraceptive administration can provide us with useful information about the mechanism of the increased risk of thromboembolism. This is of particular interest in relation to evidence that
the use of the newer pills shows a reduction of such risk.

6.2 The Coagulation-Fibrinolysis Balance

In haemostasis, the presence of fibrin is temporary and its formation
and dissolution is controlled by two counteracting mechanisms: the
coagulation and fibrinolytic mechanism. Ideally, the balance between
these two mechanisms ensures that fibrin is formed and is temporarily
present in appropriate amounts for the required time and at the appropriate places to fulfil its function in haemostatic plugging and tissue repair.

Disturbances in this balance can be due to disequilibrium between
the two systems, which in turn can be caused by disequilibrium between the activating and inhibitory mechanisms within each process.
Therefore our discussion concerns the evaluation of activation and inhibition of coagulation and the activation and inhibition of fibrinolysis.
(These four categories are shown in Fig. 1 as four parts of a circle.)

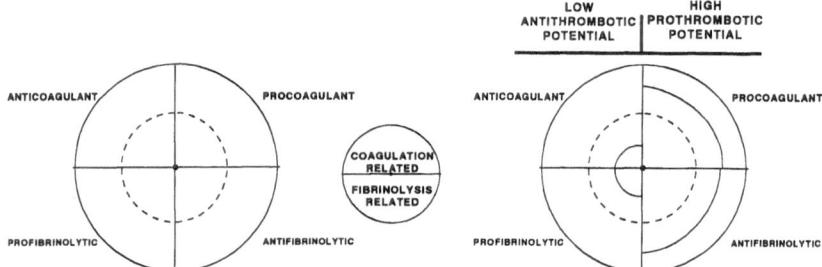

Fig. 1. a Schematic representation of the balances between coagulation and fibrinolysis (*upper* and *lower part* of the *circle*, respectively) and between activating and inhibiting factors within each system (*left* and *right parts* of the *half
circles*). The *dotted line* represents equilibrium. **b** Disequilibrium with all aspects out of balance in the direction of a prothrombotic state

6.3 Lessons from Studies on Familial Thrombophilia

Several studies in the late 1980s have addressed the problem of familial thrombophilia with the striking outcome of a prevalence equal to or even higher than the well-known familial bleeding disorders. In the Netherlands, estimates of the prevalence of familial bleeding disorders and thrombophilia are 1:15 000 and 1:3000 respectively (Bertina 1988; Engesser 1988).

One example of the studies referred to above is the Leiden Thrombophilia Study which ran from 1984 to 1988 (Engesser 1988). In this study, 37 Dutch hospitals participated in recruitment, resulting in 113 probands with a personal as well as a family history of thrombosis and 90 with only a personal history, but with a first event before the age of 40 years. The first event in probands occurred on average at age 28.3 ± 9.8 years (average for males and females; Engesser 1988). From the 93 females in the study 26 had experienced the first event while on low-dose oestrogen OCs. In comparison in the Netherlands (1988) 56.2% of the women aged 25–29 took OCs and so did 31.0% of the women of 30-34 years. This does not indicate an over-representation of OC users in the probands with heritable thrombophilia with an early onset of the clinical events.

It is important to note that attempts to identify the cause of the familial thrombophilia were only partially successful. As indicated in a schematic example in Fig. 2, the inheritance of thrombosis in the families indicated a simple mendelian autosomal dominant mode of inheritance.

This indicates that one single haemostasis factor was responsible for the problem, and with 18 assays available, in 1988, a search was carried out to identify the factor. As well as identifying deficiencies in antithrombin III ($n = 5$), protein C ($n = 13$), protein S ($n = 15$) and dysfibrinogenaemia ($n = 2$), a plasminogen deficiency and possible defects related to elevated HRG ($n = 10$), a large number of cases remained unexplained (59%). It had to be concluded that, despite the use of the majority of tests of known factors, laboratory analysis does not yet enable us to identify the individual factor(s) that is/are responsible for these problems in familial thrombophilia.

Such lack of success is, of course, partly due to the fact that coagulation and fibrinolysis are local processes and that local factors can contribute to a significant extent. The laboratory analysis utilises circu-

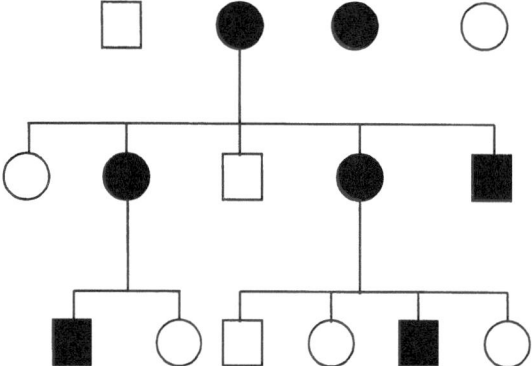

Fig. 2. Schematic example of familial thrombosis in a family with apparent mendelian inheritance and a suggestion of a heterozygosity in a single factor as the cause. Many of such families were observed in the Leiden Thrombophilia Study (Engesser 1988). *Filled circles* or *squares* are affected members of the family

lating blood and obviously misses many/all of the local aspects. What it does clearly tell us, however, is that laboratory diagnosis is insufficient and we should be modestly optimistic only about understanding the effects of the OCs on haemostasis.

6.4 Effects of OCs and Single Factor Deficiencies

From the known single factor deficiencies related to familial thrombophilia the effects of OCs on blood levels are known (Gevers Leuven et al. 1987; Jespersen et al. 1990; Task Force on Oral Contraceptives 1991; Table 1)

The effects of OCs on plasminogen (increase) and on histidine-rich glycoprotein (HRG; decrease) do not, at least, aggravate the abnormality that is associated with thrombophilia. The effect on protein C appears to be a small increase or none at all. Previous formulations of OCs did reduce antithrombin III activity and such a reduction could have been detrimental to carriers of a deficiency. Recent formulations, however, only have a minor impact, if at all, on antithrombin III blood

Table 1. Effects of oral contraceptives on factors known to be involved in familial thrombophilia

	Thrombophilia	OC effect
Antithrombin III	-	-
Protein C	-	(No effect) +
Protein S	-	-
Plasminogen	-	+
(HRG)	+	-

OC, oral contraceptives; *HRG,* histidine-rich glycoprotein; +, increase; -, decrease

Table 2. Effects of two oral contraceptives on total protein S antigen

Patients (*n*)	Before (%)	During (%)	Formulation
10*	102 ± 9	83 ± 10	30 μg ethinyl estradiol and 75 μg gestodene
9*	102 ± 14	83 ± 12	20 μg ethinyl estradiol and 150 μg desogestrel

Values are mean ± standard deviation. Data are from Jespersen et al. (1990).
*$p < 0.01$

levels. This change in the effect of newer OCs on blood levels of antithrombin III coincides with a change in the risk of thromboembolic disease and therefore antithrombin III is a likely candidate for explaining such a change. This is, however, only relevant in individuals with a low level of antithrombin III already, which would constitute a minor proportion of the population.

The lowering effects on the total amount of protein S is also observed in newer OCs. As shown in Fig. 3, in one of our studies (Gevers Leuven et al. 1990) with low-dose oestrogen pills and recent progestogens (GTD-EE = 75 μg gestodene and 30 μg ethinyl estradiol; DSG-EE = 150 μg desogestrel and 30 μg ethinyl estradiol) protein S was reduced equally by both formulations.

Similarly, as indicated in Table 2, the reduction of ethinyl estradiol to 20 μg did not result in disappearance of a reduction in protein S.

It can be concluded that reduction in protein S blood levels is also a consequence of recent formulations. This might be relevant, since hete-

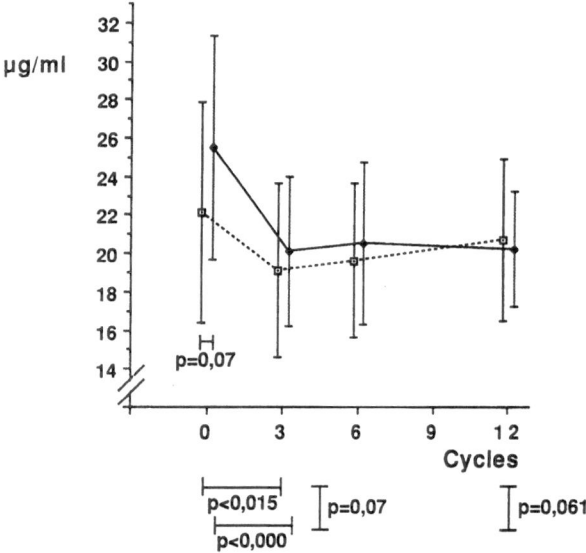

Fig. 3. Mean protein S total antigen values (± SD) (*ordinate*) in women before (*cycle 0*) and during use of OCs. For details of the study see Gevers Leuven et al. (1990). The *dotted line* represents data from 32 women using GTD-EE (75 µg gestodene and 30 µg ethinyl estradiol); the *solid line* from 28 women using DSG-EE (150 µg desogestrel and 30 µg ethinyl estradiol)

rozygous protein S deficiency constitutes a risk for thrombophilia (Engesser et al. 1987). It should, however, be noted that the risk for clinical expression of the heterozygous state for protein S showed a tendency of preference for males (Engesser et al. 1987). Furthermore, in the case of protein S, the effects of OCs on other factors that modulate protein S function, such as C4b-binding protein, should also be taken into account (Jespersen et al. 1990).

From the unknown, putative single factor deficiencies that form the basis for the familial thrombophilia in the nonexplained families (59%) we cannot judge whether or not effects of OCs further aggravate the deficiency and contribute to a risk of thromboembolic disease in this category. Taking the prevalence of familial thrombophilia as a whole (1:3000, males + females), and assuming an increase of risk by OC use

in all cases this would reflect on maximally 17 women among 100 000 users. By such a mechanism the use of OC might constitute a risk for a small group of women. The practice of using familial thrombophilia as a contraindication for OC use, however, reduces this problem.

6.5 Effects of OCs in Relation to Longitudinal Variability in Plasma Levels

Longitudinal variability in plasma concentrations differs between haemostasis variables. Some are more sensitive to day-to-day lifestyle characteristics than others. For the above-mentioned factors involved in familial thrombophilia we have used data from the follow-up after OC intake (at 3, 6 and 12 months) to evaluate the longitudinal fluctuation. We expressed the variation at these three sampling moments as standard deviation (SD_{ind}) of the individual mean value, which, as well as methodological imprecision, also includes the biological fluctuations.

As evident from Table 3, the longitudinal fluctuations are substantial. As is also indicated in Fig. 4, individuals can vary strongly in the degree of fluctuation. It can be envisaged that strong fluctuation pro-

Table 3. Variability during oral contraceptive use in plasma levels of some factors

Factor	Variability (%)
Antithrombin III	5.2 ± 3.4
Protein C	9.2 ± 5.3
Protein S	8.7 ± 6.3
Plasminogen	7.8 ± 5.4

The variability is expressed in each individual by the SD_{ind} in the individual mean value of sampling after 3, 6 and 12 months of oral contraceptive (OC) use. The data are the means of the SD_{ind} (± SD) in 58 women, expressed as a percentage of the mean pre-OC value of each variable for the whole group. The study used two pills with equal effect: 75 μg gestodene and 30 μg ethinyl estradiol; 150 μg desogestrel and 30 μg ethinyl estradiol, as reported in Gevers Leuven et al. (1990)

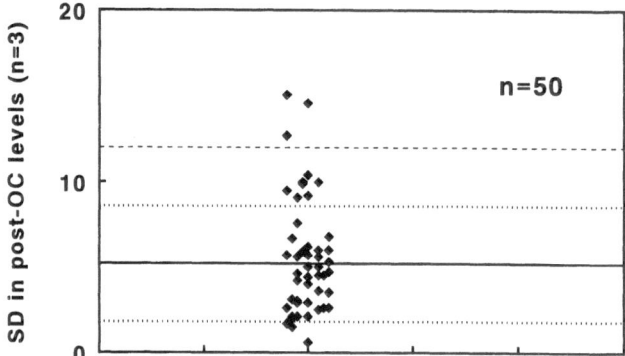

Fig. 4. Fluctuations of antithrombin III levels during oral contraceptive use. Individual fluctuations in antithrombin III expressed as SD_{ind} of the individual mean value from three sampling moments (t = 3, 6, 12 months) during oral contraceptive use (data taken from Gevers Leuven et al. (1990)). The *solid line* represents the mean; the *dotted lines* + 1 SD and + 2 SD

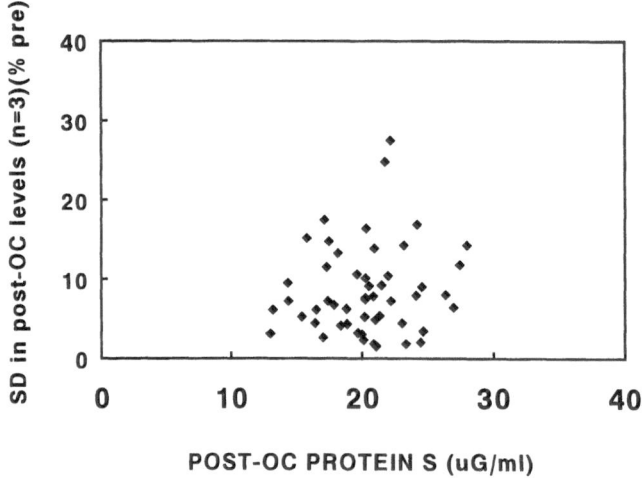

Fig. 5. Fluctuations in protein S total antigen plasma concentrations during oral contraceptive use in relation to the plasma concentration. (See legend to Fig. 4.) The SD_{ind} (*ordinate*) is expressed as a percentage of each individual plasma concentration during oral contraceptive use

vides another mechanism for creating temporary risk situations with low levels of critical factors such as antithrombin III, especially when the OC also induced a systematic reduction in such a factor such as for protein S.

An interesting question is whether the fluctuations are related to the actual plasma concentrations and whether individuals with low levels might show a reduced fluctuation or not. We evaluated this aspect for protein S, which still shows a reduction in plasma concentration even with the latest generations of OCs. As shown in Fig. 5, no clear relation between plasma level and fluctuation is apparent.

6.6 Multifactorial Risk of Thrombophilia and Multifactorial Effects of OCs

In studies on consecutive cases of thrombosis, only a small proportion relates to familial thrombophilia and to identifiable deficiencies in single (known) factors (Heyboer et al. 1990). The majority of cases are thought to be due to a multifactorial cause of the disease. One such case might be a group of persons with a pattern in multiple factors determining the potential of coagulation and fibrinolysis that causes the balance to be shifted to a prothrombotic phenotype (see Fig. 1B).

Figure 6 shows that within a given population, the status of the balance in haemostasis might range from a bleeding phenotype to a thrombotic phenotype. An arbitrary proportion may be designated as a risk category for each situation. The familial cases, of course, belong to these categories.

The many studies on effects on blood levels of individual factors of coagulation and fibrinolysis show a general pattern of an increased potential in both coagulation and in fibrinolysis. The effects include increases in procoagulant factors such as factors VII, IX and X and increases in plasminogen and decreases in the fibrinolysis inhibitors HRG and plasminogen activator inhibitor 1 (PAI-1) (see Gevers Leuven et al. 1987; Jespersen et al. 1990; Task Force on Oral Contraceptives 1991). It is possible that a procoagulant change and a profibrinolytic change balance each other.

In general, the effects of OCs on haemostatic variables are considered relatively small (note: see remarks on t-PA and PAI-1 below)

Cees Kluft et al.

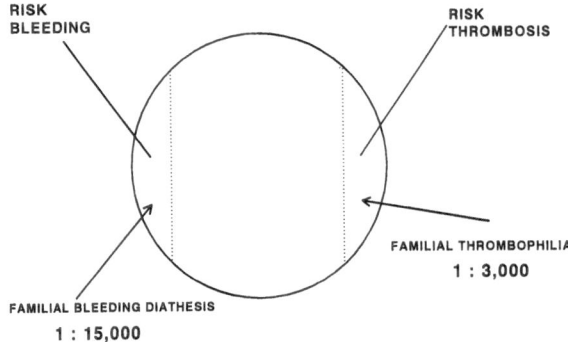

Fig. 6. Schematic subdivision of the population according to the balance in hemostasis. Two extreme situations predisposing to bleeding (*left*) or thrombosis (*right*) can be indicated. These categories harbour the cases of familial bleeding diathesis and familial thrombophilia, respectively. The proportion of the groups indicated by the *dotted line* is not proportional to the (unknown) reality

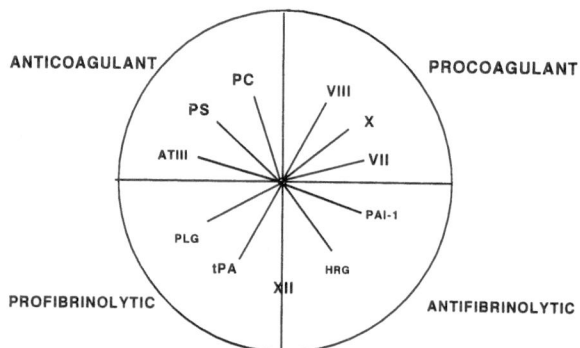

Figure 7. Specification of the factors used in the strategy of analysis used in Figs. 8 and 9. The *centre* of the *star* equals for each variable the minimum of the distribution of values in the group at a certain time. The *periphery* represents the maximum of the range. See text. *ATIII*, antithrombin III; *PS*, protein S; *PC*, protein C; *PLG*, plasminogen; *tPA*, tissue-type plasminogen activator; *PAI-1*, plasminogen activator inhibitor; *HRG*, histidine-rich glycoprotein; *VII*, *VIII*, *X*, *XII*, coagulation factors

and it seems unlikely that effects on the balance in haemostasis will bring individuals of the middle category (Fig. 6) into a state of risk. We should concentrate on the question of whether we aggravate the risk for those individuals who are assigned to the arbitrary risk category at baseline, i.e. those in whom the haemostatic balance deviates more obviously from the population mean.

Stimulated by an earlier observation that "no correlations were observed between the individual changes in fibrinolytic parameters and coagulation parameters" (Gevers Leuven et al. 1987) we tried to analyse the multifactorial aspect as outlined below.

As indicated in Fig. 7, data of individual factors of haemostasis were plotted in a circle. The factors were ordered according to categories and in quadrants, as explained in Fig. 1. The radius for each factor spanned the range of values observed in a study on 60 healthy females participating in the study (Gevers Leuven et al. 1990). Figure 8 shows a selection of five individuals (not using OCs) showing part of the variability in individual make up in haemostasis. Only one case (right, bottom case in Fig. 8, = no. 17 of the project) gave us the impression of a deviating balance, but no clear deviations such as in Fig. 1B were observed. In Fig. 9 two examples of the pattern following OCs use for 3, 6 and 12 months are given. It illustrates the observation in the whole group that the individual pattern upon use of OCs remains essentially congruent with the pattern before OC use. The variation between individuals is larger than the effect induced by OC use and spontaneous longitudinal fluctuation are sometimes larger.

This analysis supports our view that aggravation may occur only in a minority of the OC users in whom predisposition for thrombophilia was present. Such cases with a predisposition were not clearly observed in our series of individuals ($n = 60$), which concurs with the low frequency of thromboembolic complications of OC use. To further evaluate the situation, it is suggested that an analysis be carried out in individuals who develop thrombosis during OC use and to try to identify, using the above approach, possible patterns which relate to the risk and which may constitute a predisposition.

Although the effects of the newer generations of OCs on haemostatic variables are generally considered to be moderate/minor, it should be noted that the effects on tissue-type plasminogen activator (t-PA) and PAI-1 blood concentrations are substantial (Gevers Leuven et al.

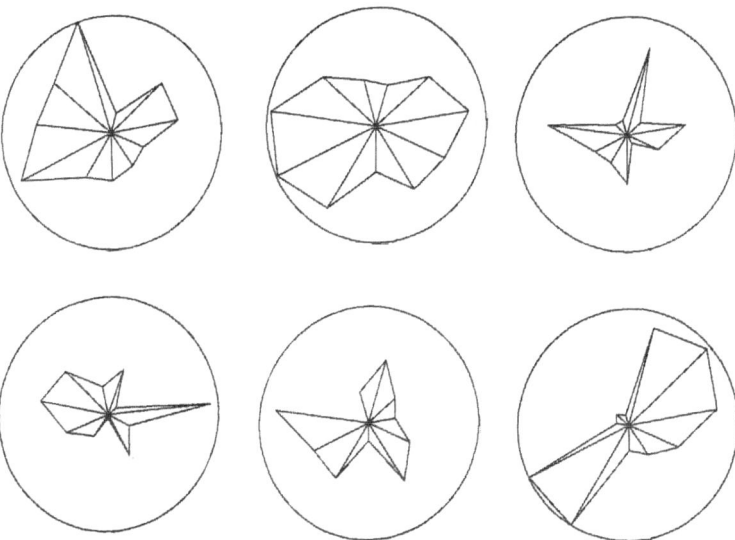

Fig. 8. *Star-plot* presentation of individual patterns of hemostasis (see Fig. 7) in six examples. Case 6 (*right, bottom*) represents an example with the most deviating pattern seen among 60 individuals, who tend towards a prothrombotic situation

1990). Since t-PA probably originates exclusively from the endothelium and PAI-1 might also reside there, this suggests a major impact on the endothelium. It is puzzling that in vitro experiments have failed to show any effect caused by steroids (Kooistra et al. 1990). An alternative explanation might be a change in clearance in the liver of both t-PA and PAI-1, or a complex between t-PA and PAI-1 (Otter et al. 1992). It can be concluded that we do not yet know the mechanism of one of the major effects of OCs in haemostasis, possibly involving the endothelium, which is a major player in the mainly local processes of coagulation and fibrinolysis.

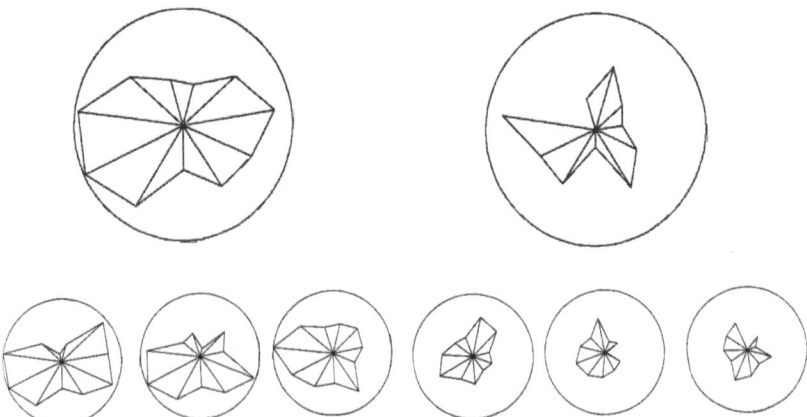

Fig. 9. Examples of effects of oral contraceptive use in two individuals according to analysis specified in Fig. 7 and the text. The *large circle* represents the pretreatment value; the *three small circles* represent the situation during oral contraceptive use and after 3, 6 and 12 months, respectively

6.7 Changes in Turnover Products
of Coagulation and Fibrinolysis Induced by OCs

The question of whether or not the changes in potential of the coagulation and fibrinolytic systems mentioned above have any clinically relevant effect can be partially evaluated by recent new methodology.

These methodologies involve the analysis of variables of the on-going action in the systems. The products of these actions, such as small peptides that are split off or truncated, or complexed molecules can be detected nowadays with specific and sensitive immunoassays frequently based on the use of specific monoclonal antibodies. Thus, it has been established, as originally proposed by Astrup (1958), that a low degree of activity in the haemostatic processes occurs continuously. This activity is evidenced by a low level of its products in blood.

We thus have the opportunity to evaluate to what extent a change in blood levels of factors, as discussed above, has an impact on the dynamics of the coagulation and fibrinolytic system in this continuous turnover. This continuous turnover can be due to either a continuous degree of activation and/or a progress "report" of daily wear and tear. As shown for congenital deficiencies, in about 25% of cases the deficiency reports itself in this way (Mannucci et al. 1992).

There are a number of reports about the effects of recent OCs on turnover products (see Abbate et al. 1990; Winkler et al. 1991). These reports indicate that (1) there is no significant effect on platelets evidenced by absence of changes in β-thromboglobulin; (2) that an effect on coagulation can occur resulting in an increase in fibrin peptide A (FPA) and/or thrombin-antithrombin III complexes (TAT); and (3) that an effect on fibrinolysis can occur resulting in increased fibrin degradation products (FDPs). In one study it was observed that an increase in both TAT and FDP did not, however, change the ratio TAT/FDP suggesting the maintenance of a balance (Gram et al. 1990).

These studies should/will in future be extended with a more sophisticated analysis of turnover products, to include, notably, more coagulation and fibrinolysis products with the intention of judging more precisely the changes that take place.

The above studies combined with an analysis of changes in the potential or levels of factors will enable us to understand more completely the impact of OCs on multiple factors of haemostasis. Potentially, this approach allows us to identify subjects with a high sensitivity to the induced changes and possibly to target those at increased risk of thromboembolic disease. This will, however, be of very limited practical value for identifying individuals at risk.

Some practical value may lie in directing the development of new OC formulations with as limited an impact on haemostasis as possible. In a recent consensus development meeting such a formulation was identified as a desired one (Consensus Development Meeting 1990) as long as we do not know how to interpret the multiple induced changes.

6.8 Concluding Remarks

Our opportunities for identifying individuals at risk for thromboembolic diseases by laboratory analysis are limited to a defined set of congenital deficiencies which mostly express themselves as familial thrombophilia. Exclusion of individuals with a family history of thromboembolic disease from OC use appears to be the only practical strategy for reducing risk at present.

References

Abbate R, Pinto S, Rustagno C, Bruni V, Rosati D, Mariani G (1990) Effects of long-term gestodene-containing oral contraceptive administration on hemostasis. Am J Obstet Gynecol 163:424-430

Astrup T (1958) The haemostatic balance. Thromb Diath Haemorrh 2:347-357

Bertina RM (1988) Prevalence of hereditary thrombophilia and the identification of genetic risk factors. Fibrinolysis 2 (suppl 2):7-13

Consensus Development Meeting: metabolic aspects of oral contraceptives of relevance for cardiovascular diseases. Am J Obstet Gynecol 162:1335-1337

Engesser L (1988) Disorders of blood coagulation and fibrinolysis. Thesis, Leiden

Engesser L, Broekmans AW, Briët E, Brommer EJP, Bertina RM (1987) Hereditary protein S deficiency: clinical manifestations. Ann Intern Med 106:677-682

Gevers Leuven JA, Kluft C, Bertina RM, Hessel LW (1987) Effects of two low-dose oral contraceptives on circulating components of the coagulation and fibrinolytic systems. J Lab Clin Med 109:631-636

Gevers Leuven JA, Kluft C, Dersjant-Roorda MC, Harthoorn-Lasthuizen EJ, Peters FPAMN, Bernsen MJ, Helmerhorst FM (1990) Changes in coagulation and fibrinolysis variables during use of two oral contraceptives containing the same dose of ethinyl estradiol and either gestodene or desogestrel. In: Elstein M (Ed) Current status of oral contraception and new developments. Advances in Contraception 6 suppl:69-73

Gram J, Munkvad S, Jespersen J (1990) Enhanced generation and resolution of fibrin in women above the age of 30 years using oral contraceptives low in estrogen. Am J Obstet Gynecol 163:438-442

Heijboer H, Brandjes DPM, Sturk A, Büller HR, Ten Cate JW (1990) Deficiencies of coagulation-inhibiting and fibrinolytic proteins in outpatients with deep-vein thrombosis. N Engl J Med 323:1512-1516

Jespersen J, Petersen KR, Skouby SO (1990) Effects of newer oral contraceptives on the inhibition of coagulation and fibrinolysis in relation to dosage and type of steroid. Am J Obstet Gynecol 163:396-403

Kooistra T, Bosma PJ, Jespersen J, Kluft C (1990) Studies on the mechanism of action of oral contraceptives with regard to fibrinolytic variables. Am J Obstet Gynecol 163:404-412

Mannucci PM, Tripodi A, Bottasso B, Baudo F, Finazzi G, De Stefano V, Palareti G, Manotti C, Mazzucconi MG, Castaman G (1992) Markers of procoagulant imbalance in patients with inherited thrombophilic syndromes. Thromb Haemostas 67:200-202

Otter M, Kuiper J, Van Berkel TJC, Rijken DC (1992) Mechanisms of tissue-type plasminogen activator (t-PA) clearance by the liver. Ann New York Acad Sci, in press

Task Force on Oral Contraceptives (1991) A multicentre study of coagulation and haemostatic variables during oral contraception: variations with four formulations. Br J Obstet Gynecol 98:1117-1128

Winkler UH, Koslowski S, Oberhoff C, Schindler EM, Schindler AE (1991) Changes of the dynamic equilibrium of hemostasis associated with the use of low-dose oral contraceptives: a controlled study of cyproterone acetate containing oral contraceptives combined with either 35 or 50 μg ethinyl estradiol. Advances in Contraception 7 suppl 3:273-284

7 Can Animal Models Be Used to Predict the Hemostasiologic Effect of Steroid Hormones in Man?

Andreas Süßmilch, Rupprecht Zierz, Karsten Parczyk,
Krzystof Chwalisz, Karl-Heinrich Fritzemeier,
and Berthold Baldus

7.1 Introduction

Epidemiologic studies indicate an increased risk of thrombosis for users of oral contraceptives (OC) which is dose-dependent for the estrogen component (Böttiger et al. 1980; Melis et al. 1988; Gerstman et al. 1991). In order to evaluate this association, most clinical studies have concentrated on the assessment of plasmatic factors to demonstrate changes in the hemostatic system caused by OC.

Whereas no changes in hemostatic plasma components could be detected throughout the ovarian cycle, alterations in plasma levels of some factors of the coagulation system have been found in OC users.

The plasma levels of prothrombin, factors VII, X and XII and fibrinogen were increased. Levels of the anticoagulant AT III were decreased, and the net balance of the protein C/S system was at most slightly altered (reviewed in Mammen 1982; Beller and Ebert 1985; Bonnar and Sabra 1986; Nawroth and Ziegler 1991). Despite the fact that these changes were significantly different from the control groups, the variations (with the exception of factor VII) barely exceeded 20% and were all within the range of the normal plasma values. Nevertheless, elevated plasma levels of fibrinopeptide A (FPA) and prothrombin fragments F_{1+2} in OC users indicate a continuous activation of the coagulation cascade (Melis et al. 1984; Skjønsberg et al. 1986; Winkler et al. 1991). Fibrinolytic activity is also thought to be induced under the influence of OC use (Daly and Bonnar 1990). Changes in fibrinolytic components were shown as decreased PAI activity and subsequently enhanced tPA activity (Jespersen et al. 1990). Molecular markers of fibrinolysis (Bβ15-42 peptide, FDP, D-dimer) were shown to be elevated by up to 100% compared to control groups (Walenga et al. 1984; Winkler et al. 1991).

Although these variations in plasmatic factors can be found in OC users and therefore imply an influence of estrogens on the hemostatic system, all these markers fail to predict the risk of thrombosis in individual OC users (Nawroth and Ziegler 1991). On the other hand, it has been shown that the perfusion of whole blood from women taking OC over desendothelialized rabbit aorta in vitro results in the apposition of significantly greater thrombus mass than with blood from non-OC users (Inauen et al. 1987).

To examine these observations in more detail, we developed an estrogen-sensitive animal model of venous thrombosis to study whether the experimentally induced thrombus formation correlated with plasmatic clotting factors.

A review of the current literature of animal models of thrombosis revealed different experimental designs. Although models of arterial thrombosis are well established and mimic the pathophysiologic state in man quite well (Bush and Shebuski 1990), no standardized model of venous thrombosis has been described thus far.

According to Virchow's hypothesis (1856), which is still valid today, venous thrombosis is caused by the triad of stasis, hypercoagulability and disturbed vessel wall. The stagnation of blood flow alone

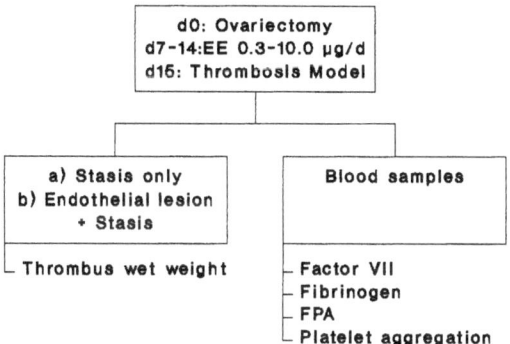

Fig. 1. Experimental design

has little effect on clotting activity; however, the combination of reduced blood flow with hypercoagulability results in thrombus formation (Wessler and Connelly 1952). In the absence of reduced blood
flow, endotoxin-induced hypercoagulability leads to a generalized fibrin generation without an overt thrombosis (Theiss and Beller 1973).
Other authors induced venous thrombosis by a combination of stasis
with an artificial surface or by endothelial damage. These studies were
performed to evaluate anti-thrombotic drugs (Reyers et al. 1980; Smith
and White 1982; Aronson and Thomas 1985; Hladovec 1986; Millet et
al. 1987).

Only a few researchers have been engaged in evaluating the effects
of steroid hormones on hemostasis in experimental animals. Using an
AV shunt model, Emms and Lewis (1985) observed an inhibition of
thrombus formation after treatment with ethinyl estradiol (EE) in rats,
whereas other authors were not able to show any effect of steroid hormones on clotting in an aortic loop model (Reel et al. 1983).

Therefore, it was of considerable importance to develop a thrombosis model which would be sensitive to sex hormones and would be
suitable to identify the mechanism by which steroid hormones influence thrombus formation. Since our attempt was primarily to determine a possible influence of OC components on venous thrombosis,
we decided to concentrate our efforts on the venous system. Our experimental design was based on the assumption that steroid hormones

cannot be considered as primary initiators of thrombosis. More likely, they may induce a hypercoagulable state and act as facilitators of thrombosis (Wessler 1989). Therefore, we combined estrogen treatment with the two other components of Virchow's triad, i.e. stasis and/or endothelial injury, to initiate thrombus formation (Fig. 1).

7.2 Methods

Animals
Wistar rats were considered as a suitable animal species, for the following reasons:

1. Necessary surgical procedures (e.g. ovariectomy, catheter implantation) were well standardized in this animal. In contrast, assays for the determination of coagulation markers are not available at present and have to be developed.
2. It was possible to evaluate the effect of cyclic changes in steroid hormones and changes on the clotting system. The effects of various synthetic and natural estrogens and progestins on the female genital tract were well established.
3. It was possible to use sufficient numbers of animals to evaluate even marginal effects.

Treatment and Blood Collection
The animals were ovariectomized 7 days prior to the experiments and treated with ethinyl estradiol (EE) 0.3-10.0 µg/day s.c. dissolved in a benzyl benzoate/castor oil (1+4) mixture for the following 7 days. Intact and ovariectomized rats served as control groups and received vehicle only.

For biochemical measurements blood was collected prior to the thrombus formation, whereas for platelet aggregation studies blood was collected after thrombus formation. Blood was carefully withdrawn through a polyethylene catheter which was inserted into the carotid artery. The anticoagulant medium (10% of the final collection volume) consisted of (a) 3.8% sodium citrate for the determination of factor VII and fibrinogen and platelet aggregation studies or (b) an inhibitor mixture of heparin (1000 IU/ml) and aprotinin (1000 KIU/ml) dissolved in 3.8% sodium citrate for the determination of FPA. Anticoagulated blood was centrifuged at 800 x g for 10 min and the plasma stored at - 80°C until performance of assays.

Thrombus Formation In Vivo
Venous thrombus formation was induced using stasis only (Reyers et al. 1980) or a combination of endothelial lesion and stasis.

Stasis Alone. Under pentobarbitone sodium anesthesia, the abdomen was opened by a midline incision. The vena cava was isolated and ligated with a cotton thread below the left renal vein. The abdomen was temporarily closed and reopened after 3 h. The vena cava was ligated for the second time at the bifurcation and the vein segment was removed, placed in 0.9% NaCl and carefully opened. If present, the thrombus was removed, washed in 0.9% NaCl and weighed immediately. The dry weight was determined after 24 h drying at room temperature.

Endothelial Lesion and Stasis. Under pentobarbitone sodium anesthesia, a balloon catheter was inserted into the femoral vein and moved into the vena cava towards the left renal vein. The balloon was inflated for endothelium denudation. Subsequently, procedures for thrombus induction were as described above.

Platelet Aggregation Ex Vivo
Platelet aggregation studies were carried out in platelet-rich plasma (PRP). Platelet count of PRP was adjusted to 600 000/μl with platelet poor plasma and diluted to 300 000 platelets/μl with 0.9% NaCl. Dose-response curves in response to ADP were obtained, measuring the increase in light transmission in an aggregometer.

Factor VII Activity
Factor VII activity was determined by a one-stage clotting assay using human factor VII-deficient plasma as the test substrate and a rat normal plasma pool for calibration.

Fibrinogen
Fibrinogen was quantified as clottable protein according to the method of Clauss (1957). Specific enzyme-linked immunosorbent assay (ELISA) techniques for the determination of rat fibrinogen and rat FPA were developed in our group.

Antigen Determination of Rat Fibrinogen

Rat fibrinogen was quantified in a sandwich ELISA using a goat IgG anti-human fibrinogen with considerable cross-reactivity towards rat fibrinogen. Streptavidin-biotin was used as the detection system. The assay was calibrated using rat fibrinogen purified by gel filtration and anion-exchange chromatography.

Quantification of Rat FPA by ELISA Technique

Synthetic rat FPA (sRtFPA) representing the 17 amino acids of native RtFPA was conjugated to keyhole limpet hemocyanin and was used for immunization to prepare rabbit IgG anti-RtFPA. The assay was based on the neutralization of the IgG binding activity towards immobilized sRtFPA by free RtFPA in the samples. Interfering fibrinogen was removed by bentonite adsorption.

Statistical Evaluation

Statistical comparisons were made using the Kruskal-Wallis test, and a probability (p) of less than 0.05 was taken as being significant.

7.3 Results

Model of Stasis Only

Applying stasis only, thrombus formation was induced in 36% of the ovariectomized animals. Treatment with EE s.c. for 7 days at doses of 0.3 and 1.0 µg/day showed no effect on the incidence of thrombus formation. A dose of 3.0 µg/day resulted in a slight increase of median thrombus weight (Table 1).

Model of Endothelial Lesion and Stasis

In this model the overall incidence of thrombus formation was 84%. In addition, thrombus wet weight was greater than in the experiments with

Fig. 2. Median wet weight of thrombi formed by endothelial denudation and ligature of the vena cava for 3 h. Ovariectomized rats were treated with ethinyl estradiol 1.0, 3.0 and 10.0 µg/day s.c. for 7 days. Control groups received vehicle only. *CI*, control intact rats; *CO*, control ovariectomized rats; *, $p <$ 0.05 vs CO. $n = 10$

Table 1. Incidence of thrombus formation and thrombus mass in ovariec-tomized rats after treatment with ethinyl estradiol in both thrombosis models

Vena cava ligation only				
	Ethinyl estradiol (µg/day)			
	0	0.3	1.0	3.0
Incidence of venous thrombosis	3/10 (30%)	3/9 (33%)	2/9 (22%)	6/10 (60%)
Median thrombus wet weight (mg)	0	0	0	0.7
Vena cava ligation + endothelial denudation				
	Ethinyl estradiol (µg/day)			
	0	0.3	1.0	3.0
Incidence of venous thrombosis	7/10 (70%)	9/9 (100%)	7/8 (88%)	8/10 (80%)
Median thrombus wet weight (mg)	8	39	22	18

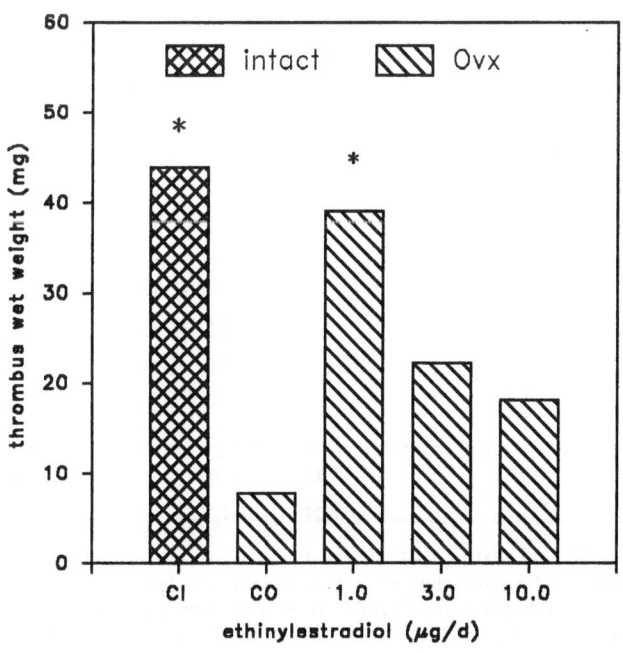

Fig. 2

stasis alone (Table 1). Thrombus formation was significantly ($p < 0.05$) suppressed by ovariectomy (7.8 mg) compared to intact animals (43.9 mg). Treatment of ovariectomized rats with 1.0 μg EE reversed this effect, whereas treatment with 3.0 or 10.0 μg EE was less effective (Fig. 2).

Platelet Aggregation

After thrombus formation with endothelial denudation and stasis, platelets from EE-treated rats showed a slight decrease in sensitivity to ADP compared with platelets from ovariectomized control rats (Fig. 3).

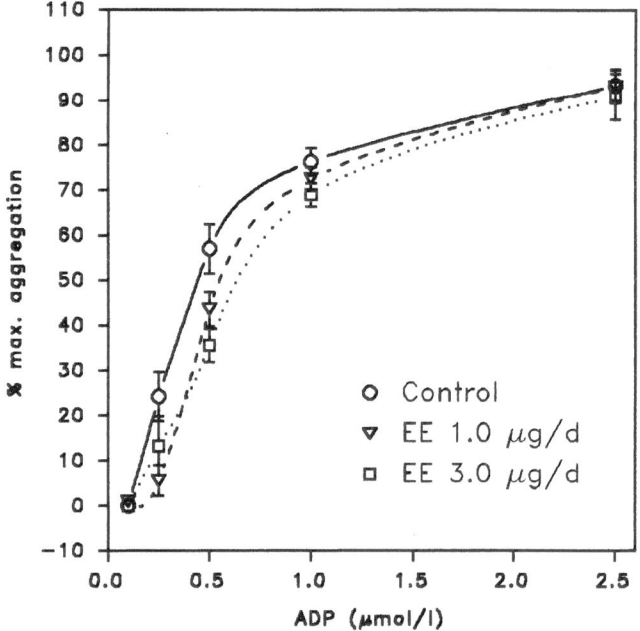

Fig. 3. ADP-induced platelet aggregation ex vivo. Ovariectomized rats were treated with 1.0 μg/day and 3.0 μg/day ethinyl estradiol (*EE*) s.c. for 7 days. The control group received vehicle only. Data are expressed as percent of maximal aggregation at 10 μmol/l ADP. *Vertical bars* represent SEM. $n = 5–7$

Factor VII

Ovariectomy led to a significant decrease in factor VII activity 14 days after surgery. In rats given 1.0 µg/day EE during the 7 days prior to ovarietomy, factor VII activity was restored, whereas the relatively high doses of 3.0 and 10.0 µg/day were not effective (Fig. 4).

Fibrinogen

A sexual dimorphism concerning fibrinogen regulation was observed. However, the plasma levels of fibrinogen in male rats remained uneffected after castration (intact males 1.35 mg/ml vs castrated males 1.31 mg/ml). On the other hand, ovariectomy of female rats significantly

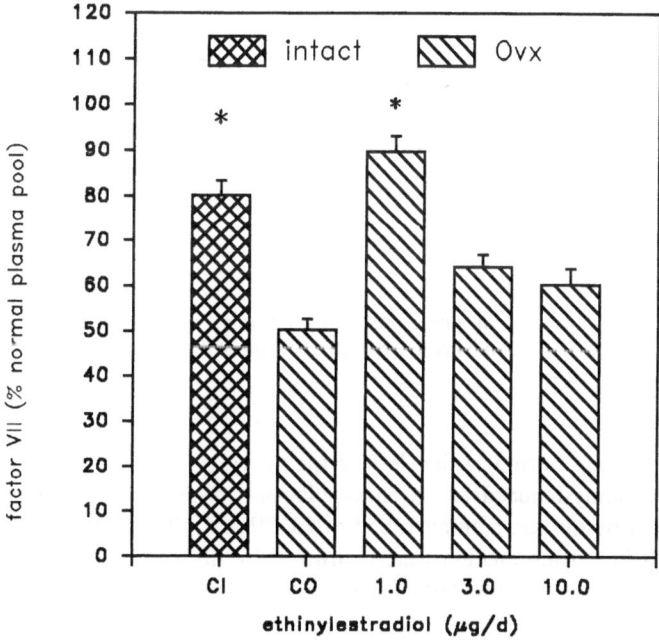

Fig. 4. Factor VII activity in female rats. Ovariectomized animals were treated with ethinyl estradiol 1.0, 3.0 and 10.0 µg/day s.c. for 7 days. Intact control rats (*CI*) and ovariectomized control rats (*CO*) received vehicle only. Data are expressed as mean ± SEM. *, $p < 0.05$ vs CO. $n = 10$

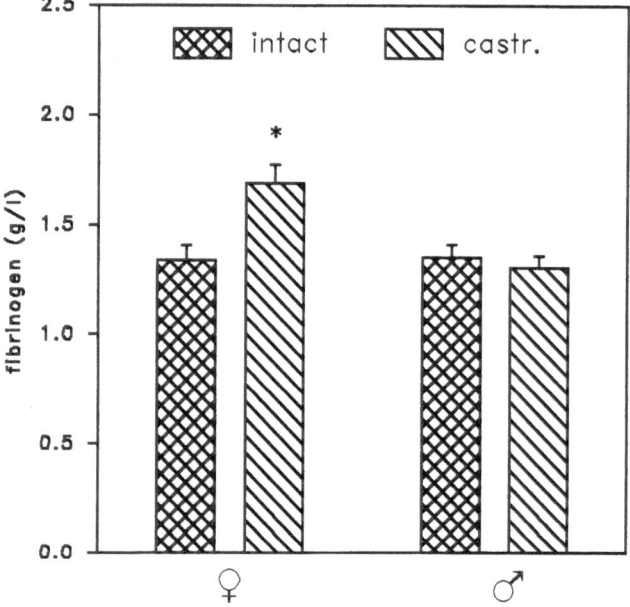

Fig. 5. Comparison of plasma fibrinogen levels of male and female rats 21 days after castration. Data are expressed as mean ± SEM. *, p < 0.05 vs intact females. $n = 10$

elevated the fibrinogen levels (1.7 mg/ml vs 1.4 mg/ml, Fig. 5). The ovariectomy-induced elevation of plasma fibrinogen levels was inhibited by the s.c. administration of EE (Fig. 6). The values obtained by ELISA determination were confirmed by fibrinogen quantification according to the method of Clauss.

Fibrinopeptide A

The values obtained for FPA plasma levels in ovariectomized or EE-substituted animals 7 days after surgery did not differ significantly from those in control animals (Fig. 7).

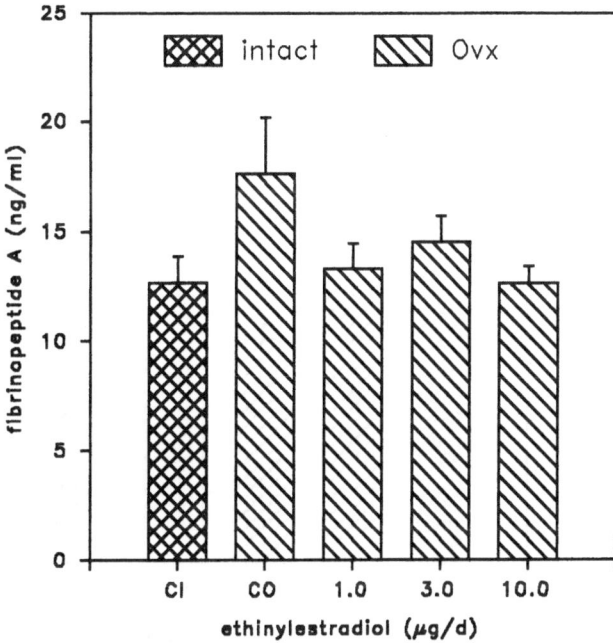

Fig. 6. Plasma fibrinogen levels of female rats. Ovariectomized animals were treated with ethinyl estradiol 1.0, 3.0 and 10.0 µg/day s.c. for 7 days. Intact control rats (*CI*) and ovariectomized control rats (*CO*) received vehicle only. Data are expressed as mean ± SEM. *, p < 0.05 vs CO. $n = 10$

7.4 Discussion

We have developed an animal model to examine the effects of sex steroids on hemostasis.

In the rat, stasis of the vena cava induced only a low incidence of thrombus formation, whereas endothelial denudation performed prior to stasis produced massive thrombi. Ovariectomy led to a significant decrease in thrombus mass which was associated with a decrease in factor VII activity; however, fibrinogen was increased. These effects could be reversed by EE.

These data indicate that experiments in which a single component of Virchow's triad, namely stasis, was used, incidence of clot forma-

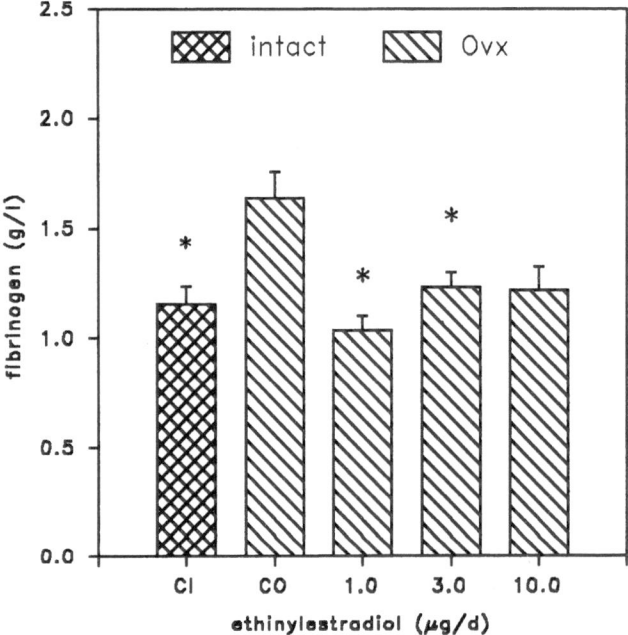

Fig. 7. Plasma FPA levels in female rats. Ovariectomized animals were treated with ethinyl estradiol 1.0, 3.0 and 10.0 μg/day s.c. for 7 days. Intact control rats (*CI*) and ovariectomized control rats (*CO*) received vehicle only. Data are expressed as mean ± SEM. $n = 10$

tion was low. The effect of EE on thrombus formation was only marginal, and probably a high number of animals would be necessary to demonstrate a significant effect of the estrogen.

It is widely accepted that the endothelium plays a physiological role in maintaining the fluidity of blood, due to its anticoagulant activity (Nawroth and Stern 1989). Endothelial denudation was used as an additional stimulus to activate hemostasis, and in combination with stasis resulted in a much higher incidence of thrombosis, in which thrombus mass was dependent on hormonal situation. Whereas ovariectomy decreased thrombus size, substitution with 1.0 μg/day EE reversed this effect. These data indicate that estrogens alone or in combination with stasis did not cause thrombosis, but clot formation was augmented and modulated by EE if endothelial damage was also present. This is in accordance with the observations of Inauen et al. (1987), that the hemostatic alterations induced by OC in combination with endothelial denudation resulted in increased fibrin formation and thrombus mass.

The increase in thrombus mass by EE was associated with a parallel increase in factor VII activity in ovariectomized rats (Figs. 2, 4). Whether the elevated factor VII activity was directly linked to the generation of large thrombi remains doubtful, as there was no correlation between factor VII activity and thrombus mass in individual animals. Nevertheless, different groups of EE-treated animals could be distinguished by their factor VII activity, and the outcome of induced thrombogenicity could be predicted in groups of experimental animals by their factor VII activity.

Elevated fibrinogen levels observed after ovariectomy were reduced to normal by EE. This effect appears to be specific and seems to be the result of an acute phase elevation of fibrinogen in response to the surgery, as FPA levels did not differ significantly between ovariectomized and control animals. A more reliable analysis of an acute inflammatory reaction would be the determination of other acute phase products besides fibrinogen. In addition, the value of FPA determinations in monitoring inflammatory or surgical events is limited due to the short half-life of FPA. The analysis of D-dimer and prothrombin fragments F_{1+2} would be useful to exclude inflammatory effects (Boisclair et al. 1990).

The low incidence of thrombus formation in our model in which stasis alone was used is in accordance with observations from epidemiologic studies which showed that thrombosis is a rare phenomenon, even with OC intake, in healthy women. Our data showing that alterations of the vessel wall are necessary to demonstrate effects of estrogens on thrombosis are also consistent with epidemiologic studies showing an increased incidence of thrombosis in OC users if they were additionally predisposed by having one or more risk factors of vascular disease (Thorogood and Vessey 1990).

In contrast to epidemiologic studies, the well-documented elevated plasma fibrinogen levels induced by OC in women could not be found in our animal model. Elevated FPA values in women using OC should be considered as an index of the hemostatic turnover. A sustained two- to threefold increase in fibrinopeptides (FPA, Bβ15-42) reflects a permanent massive activation of the coagulation and fibrinolysis systems.

During major surgery (gastric/hepatic resection), only a transient five-fold increase in FPA plasma levels has been reported (Kambayashi et al. 1990). Neither the elevation of fibrinogen nor the elevation of FPA plasma levels observed in OC users was found in our animal model. Therefore, ovariectomized rats substituted with estrogens apparently do not reflect the clinical state of women using OC in this respect. The effects of steroid hormones on intact female rats are currently under investigation.

7.4.1 Further Perspectives:
The Regulation of Coagulation Factors by Sex Steroids

The observation that estrogens modulate the activity of factor VII in the rat raises the question of the molecular mechanism underlying this effect. In general, steroids act by binding to and activating their receptors, which act as transactivating factors. The hormone-receptor complexes are able to bind to specific promoter or enhancer regions of target genes (Beato 1989). Such regions (estrogen-responsive elements, EREs) have been described for two genes for blood plasma proteins. The vitellogenin gene is estrogen-dependently expressed in the liver of oviparous animals (Klein-Hitpaß et al. 1986), and recently it has been shown by Feldmer et al. (1991) that the promoter of the rat angiotensinogen gene carries an ERE-like element. The EREs of other estrogen-dependent plasma proteins such as sex hormone-binding globulin, corticosterone-binding globulin or clotting factors have not yet been identified. Furthermore, it is not clear whether these genes are regulated directly by estrogens via the hepatic estrogen receptor or indirectly by other (estrogen-modulated) hormones such as growth hormone, prolactin, thyroxine or glucocorticoids. To answer this question, the use of tissue culture models allowing a direct incubation of isolated liver cells with different hormones might be helpful. However, our own experiments with the human liver hepatoma cell line HepG2 showed that the effects of estrogens in this system are barely more than moderate. We have been unable to demonstrate detectable amounts of estrogen receptor in these cells, in contrast to normal human liver tissue (unpublished observations, Burch et al. 1988).

We are now studying the expression of several blood plasma proteins in the liver under estrogen treatment. Furthermore, we will use primary cultures of rat liver hepatocytes to examine whether these genes which are estrogen-sensitive in vivo are regulated directly by estrogens.

At present we have studied the effects of estrogens on angiotensinogen and on insulin-like growth factor 1 (IGF-1) in the liver. The data for coagulation factors are not available yet. In accordance with others (Ganten et al. 1990), we found a dose-dependent increase in angiotensinogen plasma levels in the rat in vivo as well as in cultivated hepatocytes (data not shown) after treatment with EE. Furthermore, we observed that IGF-1 was down-regulated in vivo on the protein level as well as on the mRNA level by EE. Comparable results have been reported by Murphy and Friesen (1988). Our preliminary experiments on the effect of estrogens on IGF-1 production in vitro indicate that the estrogen modulation of this protein might be regulated indirectly by a so far unknown mechanism.

7.5 Conclusion

Our data indicate that endogenous or exogenous estrogens modulate thrombogenesis if the vessel wall is injured. However, the mechanism of action of the estrogens remains unclear. In particular, it is not known whether this represents a direct or indirect effect of estrogens.

Acknowledgements. We thank C. Dobrindt for expert technical assistance and Dr. W. Witt, M. Fredrich, Dr. P. Verhallen, Dr. F. McDonald, Prof. G. Stock and Dr. P.P. Nawroth for their cooperation, inspiring discussions and critical reading of the manuscript.

References

Aronson DL, Thomas DP (1985) Experimental studies on venous thrombosis: effect of coagulants, procoagulants and vessel contusion. Thromb Haemost 54: 866-870

Beato M (1989) Gene regulation by steroid hormones. Cell 56: 335-344

Beller FK, Ebert C (1985) Effects of oral contraceptives on blood coagulation: a review. Obstet Gynecol Surv 40: 425-436

Boettiger LE, Boman G, Eklund G, Westerholm B (1980) Oral contraceptives and thromboembolic disease: effects of lowering oestrogen content. Lancet 5: 1097-1101

Boisclair MD, Ireland H, Lane DA (1990) Assessment of hypercoagulable states by measurement of activation fragments and peptides. Blood Rev 4: 25-40

Bonnar J, Sabra AM (1986) Oral contraceptives and blood coagulation. J Repr Med 31: 551-556

Burch JBE, Evans MI, Friedman TM, O'Malley PJ (1988) Two functional estrogen response elements are located upstream of the major chicken vitellogenin gene. Mol Cell Biol 8: 1123-1131

Bush LR, Shebuski RJ (1990) In vivo models of arterial thrombosis and thrombolysis. FASEB J 4: 3087-3098

Clauss VA (1957) Gerinnungsphysiologische Schnellmethode zur Bestimmung des Fibrinogens. Acta Haematol 17: 237-246

Daly L, Bonnar J (1990) Comparative studies of 30 µg ethinyl estradiol combined with gestodene and desogestrel on blood coagulation, fibrinolysis and platelets. Am J Obstet Gynecol 163: 430-437

Emms H, Lewis GP (1985) The effect of synthetic ovarian hormones on an in vivo model of thrombosis in the rat. Br J Pharmacol 84: 243-248

Feldmer M, Kaling M, Takahashi S, Mullins JJ, Ganten D (1991) Glucocorticoid- and estrogen-responsive elements in the 5'-flanking region of the rat angiotensinogen gene. J Hypertens 9: 1005-1012

Ganten D, Hellmann W, Klett C, Weimar-Ehl T, Feldmer M, Hackenthal E, Ryffel GU (1990) Differential actions of steroid hormones on the expression of the angiotensinogen gene expression. Eur J Pharmacol 183: 690

Gerstman BB, Piper JM, Tomita DK, Ferguson WJ, Stadel BV, Lundin FE (1991) Oral contraceptive estrogen dose and the risk of deep venous thromboembolic disease. Am J Epidemiol 133: 32-37

Hladovec J (1986) Antithrombotics in view of thrombosis models. Thromb Res 43: 545-551

Inauen W, Baumgartner HR, Haeberli A, Straub PW (1987) Excessive deposition of fibrin, platelets and platelet thrombi on vascular subendothelium during contraceptive drug treatment. Thromb Haemost 57: 306-109

Jespersen J, Petersen KR, Skouby SO (1990) Effects of newer oral contraceptives on the inhibition of coagulation and fibrinolysis in relation to dosage and type of steroid. Am J Obstet Gynecol 163: 396-403

Kambuyashi J, Sakon M, Yokato M, Shiba E, Kawasaki T, Mori T (1990) Activation of coagulation and fibrinolysis during surgery, analyzed by molecular markers. Thromb Res 60: 157-167

Klein-Hitpaß L, Schorpp M, Wagner U, Ryffel GU (1986) An estrogen-responsive element derived from the 5' flanking region of the Xenopus vitellogenin A2 gene functions in transfected human cells. Cell 46: 1053-1061

Kooistra T, Bosma PJ, Jespersen J, Kluft C (1990) Studies on the mechanism of action of oral contraceptives with regard to fibrinolytic variables. Am J Obstet Gynecol 163: 404-413

Mammen EF (1982) Oral contraceptives and blood coagulation: a critical review. Am J Obstet Gynecol 142: 781-790

Melis GB, Fruzzetti F, Paoletti AM, Carmassi F, Fioretti P (1984) Fibrinopeptide A plasma levels during low-estrogen oral contraception treatment. Thromb Res 30: 575-583

Melis GB, Fruzetti F, Ricci C, Carmassi F, Fioretti P (1988) Oral contraceptives and venous thromboembolic disease: the effect of the oestrogen dose. Maturitas Suppl 1: 131-139

Murphy LJ, Friesen HG (1988) Differential effects of estrogen and growth hormone on uterine and hepatic insulin-like growth factor I gene expression in the ovariectomized hypophysectomized rat. Endocrinology 122: 325-332

Nawroth PP, Stern DM (1989) Das Endothel als zentrale Schaltstelle der Gerinnungskaskade. Z Kardiol 78: Suppl 6, 16-24

Nawroth PP, Ziegler R (1991) Die Antibaby-Pille als Risikofaktor einer Thrombose: sind molekulare Mechanismen bekannt? Klin Wochenschr 69: 335-339

Millet J, Theveniaux J, Pascal M (1987) A new experimental model of venous thrombosis in rats involving partial stasis and slight endothelium alterations. Thromb Res 45: 123-133

Reel JR, McKenzie JS, Collins DW, Edgren RA (1983) Steroid-induced thrombogenesis in rats. Int J Fert 28: 169-172

Reyers I, Mussoni L, Donati MB, deGaetano G (1989) Failure of aspirin at different doses to modify experimental thrombosis in rats. Thromb Res 18: 669-674

Skjønsberg OH, Kierulf P, Fagerhol MK, Godal HC (1986) Thrombin generation during collection and storage of blood. Vox Sang 50: 33-37

Smith JR, White AM (1982) Fibrin, red cell and platelet interactions in an experimental model of thrombosis. Br J Pharmacol 77: 029-033

Theiss W, Beller FK (1973) Stilbestrol-augmented disseminated intravascular coagulation in rats after infusion of endotoxin. Am J Obstet Gynecol 115: 775-782

Thorogood M, Vessey MP (1990) An epidemiologic survey of cardiovascular disease in women taking oral contraceptives. Am J Obstet Gynecol 163: 274-281

Virchow RLK (1856) Gesammelte Abhandlungen zur wissenschaftlichen Medizin. Meidinger, Frankfurt/Main

Walenga JM, Fareed J, Mariani G, Messmore HL, Bick RL, Emanuele RM (1984) Diagnostic efficacy of a simple radioimmunoassay test for fibrinogen/fibrin fragments containing the Bβ15-42 sequence. Sem Thromb Haemost 10: 252-263

Wessler S (1989) The issue of animal models of thrombosis. Ann NY Acad Sci 556: 366-370

Wessler S, Connelly MT (1952) Studies in intravascular coagulation. I. Coagulation changes in isolated venous segments. J Clin Invest 31: 1011-1014

Winkler UH, Bühler K, Oberhoff C, Koslowski S, Hölscher T, Schindler AE
(1991) Cyclic variation of haemostatic activities during the menstrual
cycle: Modulation by low dose oral contraceptives. Abstract 1262, XIII
Congress of the International Society on Thrombosis and Haemostasis,
Amsterdam

8 Estradiol and Myointimal Proliferation

Marie L. Foegh

8.1 Introduction

Epidemiological studies have shown estrogen to be beneficial in protecting women from cardiovascular disease. The continual rise in the use of estrogen in an increasing adult female population has made elucidation of the effect of estrogen on the vascular system important.

Estradiol has been shown to inhibit proliferation of primary cultures of smooth muscle cells from different species. As early as 1978, Colburn and Buonassisi showed that smooth muscle cells obtained from the rat aorta had estrogen binding sites. More recently, our own group has shown specific high affinity binding sites for estradiol in primary cultures of rat cardiac smooth muscle cells and rat cardiac endothelial cells (Bei et al., submitted).

It is generally accepted that in the normal postmenopausal women, estrogen treatment would be beneficial for protecting against osteoporosis and cardiovascular problems. However, organ transplantation presents a challenge to whether estrogen treatment should be given to postmenopausal women who have received an organ transplant. Some of the known effects of estrogen, namely, increase in macrophage function and increased immune response in some autoimmune diseases, suggest that estrogen use in postmenopausal women having an organ transplant may increase the risk of organ rejection. However, other aspects of estrogen effects, namely, increase in HDL cholesterol, may speak to a possible advantage of estrogen treatment. A major problem particularly in cardiac transplantation is accelerated coronary artery atherosclerosis. It has been described in different studies to occur in 25-80% of patients (Gao et al. 1987; Hess et al. 1987; Uretsky et al. 1987). These huge variations in incidence may depend on the intensity of patient follow up by coronary artery angiography by the different centers. In general the U.S. centers seem to report a higher incidence of accelerated cardiac transplant atherosclerosis than is seen in the European centers. In order to elucidate the possible effects of estradiol we initiated a series of studies evaluating the effect of estradiol in vivo and in vitro on vascular smooth muscle cell proliferation.

8.2 Estrogen and Accelerated Transplant Atherosclerosis

In the heterotopic cardiac transplant model in the rabbit, the allograft is placed in the neck of rabbits with an end-to-side anastomosis between the aorta and the carotid artery and the pulmonary artery and the jugular vein. In this model, both the donor and recipient rabbits are fed a 0.5% cholesterol diet 1 week prior to transplantation. The cholesterol diet is continued in the recipient until sacrifice at 5 to 6 weeks after transplantation. This diet increases the normal rabbit serum cholesterol level from 30 mg/dl to 400-600 mg/dl. The rabbits are all given cyclosporin A 10 mg/kg per day s.c. in order to prevent rejection in this strong histoincompatible model. The coronary arteries were evaluated at 3, 7, 21, and 40 days after transplantation in order to determine by histology using light microscopy and electron microscopy the evolution of the myointimal hyperplasia (Kuwahara et al. 1991). The first interesting finding was that the myointimal hyperplasia occurred under an ultrastructurally normal endothelium. Further, for the first 3 weeks, the intimal thickening consisted of mainly smooth muscle cells, but from week 3 to week 6, an increasing number of macrophages appeared in the intima. In this model of coronary artery accelerated atherosclerosis, the effect of daily treatment with 17β-estradiol 100 µg/kg per day on myointimal hyperplasia was evaluated (Foegh et al. 1987). It was found that daily treatment with estradiol significantly inhibited the myointimal hyperplasia 6 weeks after transplantation.

These studies were repeated in a different transplant model in which the abdominal aorta from the rabbit was transplanted to the neck of the recipient rabbit (Cheng et al. 1991). In this model, where the rabbit also received cyclosporine 10 mg/kg per day, the myointimal hyperplasia was evaluated by morphometry and by histology and electron microscopy 3 weeks after transplantation. Four different doses of estradiol were compared to placebo (1, 10, 100, 1000 µg/kg per day of estradiol cypionate). All four doses of estradiol had similar effects on inhibition of myointimal hyperplasia in spite of the lowest dose just maintaining serum estradiol levels at just slightly above the normal male rabbit levels, 29.6 ± 2.7 pg/ml and 21.1 ± 0.7 pg/ml, respectively. However, at the lowest dose of estradiol, macrophages appeared occasionally in the myointima whereas in the three groups receiving the higher doses of estradiol no macrophages were seen.

A further interesting finding was that in the endothelium from the transplanted aorta of the rabbits receiving the different doses of estradiol, the endothelial cell layer appeared ultrastructurally normal compared to the control group, where degenerative changes were observed in the endothelial cells. Fig. 1 shows the electron micrograph of the aorta graft from control rabbits and from rabbits receiving estradiol cypionate. The myointima of the control rabbits contains lipid laden macrophages as well as lipid laden smooth muscle cells, while the aorta from estradiol treated animals appears without macrophages and only few smooth muscle cells in the intima.

In two different models of accelerated transplant atherosclerosis, estradiol was found to inhibit myointimal hyperplasia where the lowest dose administered was 1 µg/kg per day, and the highest, 1000 µg/kg

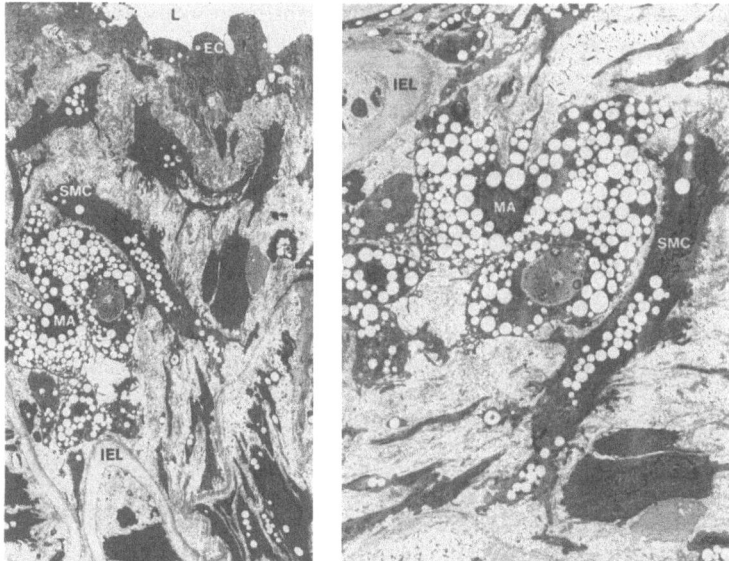

a   b

Fig. 1. a Electron micrograph of aorta graft intima shows macrophage-derived foam cells (*MA*) and vacuolized smooth muscle cells (*SMC*) in a placebo-treated rabbit (x 1200). **b** Macrophage-derived foam cell (*MA*) and vacuolized smooth muscle cell (*SMC*) in the intima of a graft from a placebo-treated rabbit (x 2000)

per day. Estradiol seems to preserve the endothelial cells and to prevent at the three highest doses the appearance of macrophages in the myointima.

8.3 Estrogen and Myointimal Hyperplasia Following Vascular Injury

The regulation of myointimal hyperplasia in accelerated transplant atherosclerosis and in arteries injured by, for example, balloon angioplasty, is very likely similar. In the balloon injured artery the endothelium is removed, whereas in the transplanted organ, the endothelium remains intact following transplantation. In spite of the differences in

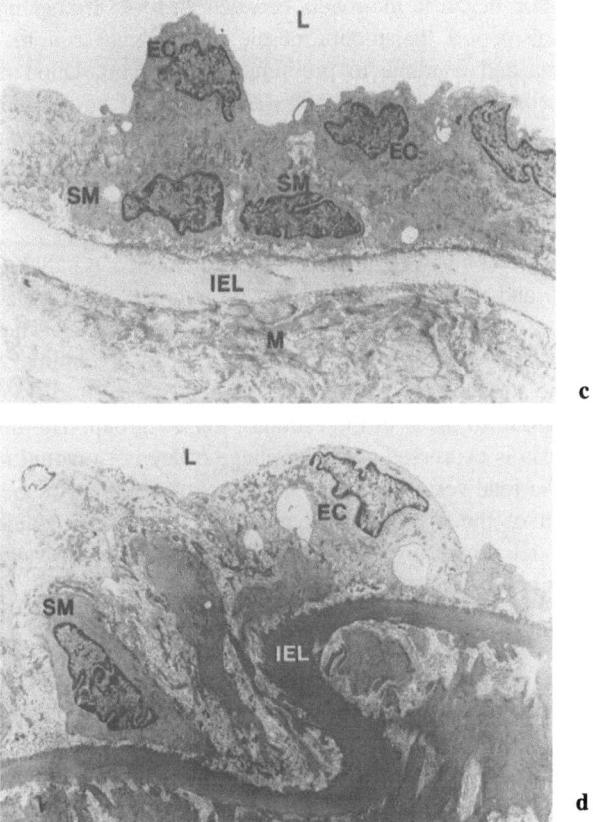

Fig. 1. c Reduced vacuolization in smooth muscle cells (*SM*) and absence of macrophages in the graft of a rabbit receiving 10 µg/kg per day estradiol cypionate (x 3000). **d** No vacuolization in smooth muscle cells (*SM*) and absence of macrophages in the graft of a rabbit receiving 100 µg/kg per day estradiol cypionate (x 3000). *L*, lumen; *EC*, endothelial cell; *IEL*, internal elastic lamina; *M*, media. (From Cheng et al. 1991)

the presence of endothelium, the mechanisms of preventing the smooth muscle cell migration and proliferation might very well be similar. Fishman et al. (1975) already observed in the rat carotid artery damaged by a balloon embolectomy catheter that the smooth muscle cell proliferation began in the media between 24 to 48 h after injury. Following this period, the smooth muscle cells migrate from the media to the intima and continue to proliferate. The accumulation of smooth muscle cells is at a maximum at 2 weeks in the rat carotid artery model. However, the intima continues thickening in that extracellular matrices are formed and the entire thickness of the intima reaches a maximum at 28 days. Using the rabbit aorta carotid artery balloon injury, we studied the effect of estrogen in preventing myointimal hyperplasia.

Fourteen rabbits were anesthetized and underwent balloon injury of the aorta and iliac arteries. The treated animals were given estradiol 100 µg/kg per day as in the cardiac transplant studies. The estrogen treated rabbits exhibited significant decrease in myointimal hyperplasia. In the aorta the myointimal thickness decreased from 18.6% in the control group to 5.7% in the estradiol treated group. The myointimal hyperplasia is expressed as a percentage of area of myointimal hyperplasia over total vessel area. The mechanisms of action for the estradiol inhibition of the myointimal hyperplasia was further studied in the same model, where thymidine uptake was used as a measurement for cell proliferation (Howell et al., submitted).

8.4 ^{3}H-Thymidine Uptake in the Rabbit Iliac Vessels Following Balloon Injury

A series of rabbits underwent balloon injury of the aorta. The animals were treated with estradiol at the same doses as in the previous experiment. At 48 h following the balloon injury, radioactive thymidine was injected intravenously, and the animals were sacrificed 72 h later. It was found that estradiol inhibited significantly the thymidine uptake in the aorta (Howell et al., submitted).

8.5 Sex Differences in Estradiol Inhibition of Thymidine Uptake

In order to study whether differences in inhibition of myointimal hyperplasia following balloon injury would occur in the rabbit balloon injury model, an experiment was carried out in both male and female

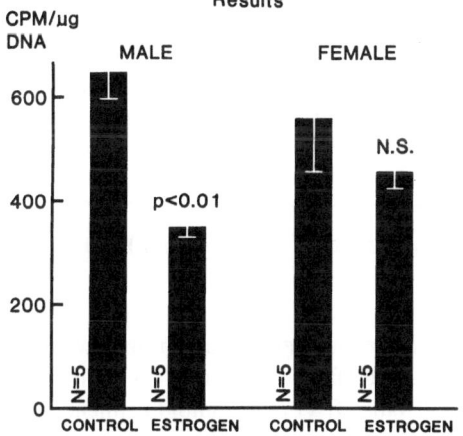

Fig. 2. Results of a ^{3}H-thymidine uptake in vivo/in vitro myointimal hyperplasia-rabbit. Male and female rabbits underwent balloon injury of the abdominal aorta. Both the male and female animals were divided into a control group and a group receiving estradiol cypionate 100 μg/kg per day. The animals were sacrificed at 72 h and the thymidine uptake was determined in vitro in the aorta. The ^{3}H-thymidine uptake is expressed as counts per minute (CPM) per microgram DNA

rabbits who underwent balloon injury. The animals were treated with estradiol cypionate, 100 μg/kg per day, or placebo. The rabbits were injected with radiolabeled thymidine 48 h after balloon injury and sacrificed 72 h after balloon injury. It was found that estradiol significantly inhibited the thymidine uptake in the male rabbits and also inhibited thymidine uptake in the female rabbits, but in the female rabbits the inhibition was not significantly different from the control group (Fig. 2).

These in vivo studies showed that estradiol inhibits myointimal hyperplasia in a model of balloon injury and that the inhibitory effect of estradiol is exerted on the smooth muscle cell proliferation as determined by thymidine uptake.

8.6 Estrogen Inhibition of In Vitro Thymidine Uptake in Pig Coronary Arteries

Pig coronary arteries were incubated in vitro with different concentrations of estradiol, as well as with solvent alone. It was found that estrogen inhibited in vitro myointimal hyperplasia (thymidine uptake) in pig coronary arteries in vitro (Vargas et al., In Press).

8.7 Estrogen Inhibition of Myointimal Hyperplasia in Vein Grafts

Human coronary saphenous vein bypass grafts develop atherosclerosis more readily than do grafts from the internal mammary artery. In this study, we evaluated the effect of estradiol treatment on the myointimal hyperplasia determined by morphometry in the jugular vein which was interpositioned in the carotid artery. The studies were carried out in normal cholesterolemic rabbits in whom a jugular vein was interpositioned end-to-end in the carotid artery. Estrogen was found to have no effect on the myointimal hyperplasia found 21 days following surgery. In order to further confirm the initial observation that estradiol had no effect on venous myointimal hyperplasia in vivo, we also studied saphenous veins from female patients and the femoral vein from dogs. Ring segments of the veins were incubated in vitro in tissue culture media in order to evaluate thymidine uptake in the presence of estradiol. It was found both in the dog and in the human saphenous vein that estradiol had no effect on thymidine uptake, unlike forskolin, which was shown to inhibit thymidine uptake (Calcagno et al., in Press).

From the in vivo and in vitro experiments on veins from rabbits, humans and dogs, it was concluded that estrogen does not inhibit the myointimal hyperplasia in veins.

8.8 Summary

Several experimental models, both in vivo and in vitro, show that estrogen inhibits myointimal hyperplasia in the arteries of the experimental animals evaluated. In the cardiac transplant model, and aorta transplant model, the effect of estrogen may partially be expressed through maintenance of an ultrastructurally and functionally normal endothelium. The mechanisms for the inhibition can be speculated to be through an inhibition of the secondary intracellular messengers of different growth factors causing smooth muscle cell proliferation.

References

Bei M, Foegh M, Ramwell P, Clarke R (1992) Specific high affinity binding sites for 17β-estradiol in primary cultures of rat heart smooth muscle cells and rat heart endothelial cells. Circ Res (Submitted)

Calcagno D, Bei M, Ross SA, Klein A, Foegh ML (1992) Effects of estrogen on vein grafts. J Cardiovasc Surgery (In Press)

Cheng L, Kuwahara M, Jacobsson J, Foegh ML (1991) Inhibition of myointimal hyperplasia and macrophage infiltration by estradiol in aorta allografts. Transplantation 52:967-972

Colburn P, Buonassisi V (1978) Estrogen-binding sites in endothelial cell cultures. Science 201(4358):817-819

Fishman JA, Ryan GB, Karnowsky MJ (1975) Endothelial regeneration in the rat carotid artery and the significance of endothelial denudation in the pathogenesis of myointimal thickening. Lab Invest 32:339

Foegh M, Khirabadi BS, Nakanishi T, Vargas R, Ramwell PW (1987) Estradiol protects against experimental cardiac transplant atherosclerosis. Transplant Proc 19 (Suppl 5):90-95

Gao SZ, Schroeder JS, Alderman EL, Hunt SA, Silverman JF, Wiederhold V, Stinson EB (1987) Clinical and laboratory correlates of accelerated coronary artery disease in the cardiac transplant patient. Circulation 76 (Suppl V):56

Hess ML, Hastillo A, Thompson JA, Sansonetti DJ, Zentpetery SS, Barnhart G, Lower RR (1987) Lipid mediators in organ transplantation: Does cyclosporine accelerate coronary atherosclerosis. Transplant Proc 19 (Suppl 5):71-73

Howell M, Asotra S, Foegh M, Ramwell P (1992) Effect of estradiol 17-β on myointimal hyperplasia after balloon injury in rabbits. Circulation Res (Submitted)

Kuwahara M, Jacobsson J, Kuwahara M, Kagan E, Ramwell PW, Foegh ML (1991) Coronary artery ultrastructural changes in cardiac transplant atherosclerosis in the rabbit. Transplantation 52:759-765

Uretsky BF, Murali S, Reddy PS, Rabin B, Lee A, Griffith BP, Hardesty RL, Trento A, Bahnson TH (1987) Development of coronary artery disease in cardiac transplant patients receiving immunosuppressive therapy with cyclosporine and prednisone. Circulation 76:827

Vargas R, Wroblewska B, Rego A, Hatch J, Ramwell PW (1992) Estradiol inhibits smooth muscle cell proliferation of pig coronary artery. J Pharmacol Exp Ther (Submitted)

9 Modulation of the Extracellular Matrix by Sex Steroids

Hermann Graf

9.1 Introduction

Steroid hormones are known to be important regulators of growth, development, maturation, and aging. It is widely accepted that sex steroids act via specific receptor proteins localized in the cytoplasm (glucocorticoid, mineralocorticoid) or in the nuclear (estrogen, progesterone) compartment. The steroid-receptor complexes tightly bind to hormone responsive elements of genes. In this way steroid hormones regulate physiological and pathophysiological processes by activating or suppressing transcription of genes under its control. Sex hormones influence organization and function of cells and tissue not only within the genital tract. Gender differences have also been found in the cardiovascular system.

9.2 Sexual Dimorphism and Vascular Structure

Thus, sex steroids seemed to determine the anatomy of the myocardium (deSimone et al. 1991), blood fluidity, and endothelium-platelet interaction (Berge et al. 1990), plasma lipoprotein pattern and content (Weidner et al. 1991), and vascular reactivity (Brizzolara et al. 1992). At any age, although to a different extent, the risk of cardiovascular disease is higher in men than in women. Hormonal changes due to hysterectomy or onset of menopause clearly alters sexual dimorphism in vascular disease. Estrogen replacement therapy has been claimed to decrease (Stampfer et al. 1985) or increase (Wilson et al. 1985) the risk of vascular disease. Ten-year follow-up from the Nurses' Health Study including over 48 000 postmenopausal women revealed that 17β-estradiol is cardioprotective (Stampfer et al. 1985). The cardiovascular risk or benefit was claimed to be closely related to the dose and potency of the estrogens (Lobo 1990).

9.3 Sex Steroids and Vascular Cell Function

The mechanism of action of sex steroids still remains to be elucidated. Immunochemically, estrogen and progesterone receptors were found in uterine arteries, suggesting that sex steroids may regulate uterine blood flow through an effect on the vessel wall (Perrot-Applanat et al. 1988). Estrogen and progesterone receptors were also found in rat aorta and expressed gender differences. Aortic progesterone receptor content could be increased by exogenous 17β-estradiol (Lin et al. 1986). The view of sex steroids acting on the vasculature is supported by earlier, more detailed investigations on the sexual dimorphism in vascular prostacyclin production (Pommerantz et al. 1980), endothelium-dependent regulation of vascular tone (Zhang et al. 1992), and in the development of raised fibrous lesions which seemed to be dependent on age and sex (Mitchell et al. 1964). Modulation of vascular responses occurred in sclerotic coronary arteries in a rabbit model (Williams et al. 1990) and even direct effects of estradiol were seen in cell culture. The proliferation of vascular smooth muscle cells is concentration dependently inhibited by estradiol (Rhee et al. 1978). In sum, vascular organization and reactivity is directly influenced by sex steroids on the level of cell differentiation, cellular organization, and vasoactive factors produced by the vasculature.

9.4 Sex Steroids and Vascular Remodeling

The influences of sex steroids on tissue remodeling are well known in respect to cervix dilatation in pregnancy and labor. It was shown that estrogens mediate collagenolysis in the guinea pig cervix (Rajabi et al. 1991). Degradation of type I collagen was demonstrated immunochemically in the dilated cervix at parturition and induction of collagenase activity could be mimicked by exogenous 17β-estradiol at physiological concentrations in the nonpregnant cervix in organ culture. The effect of estradiol was completely blocked by progesterone at high concentrations. Altered collagen structure and organization was additionally shown after estrogen treatment in the immature rat uterus (Pastore et al. 1989; Too et al. 1986). Structural changes already occurred after 1 h of treatment followed by a series of late events, including water uptake, growth, and changes in lipid and glucose metabolism. Today it is still unclear whether sex steroids are directly acting on uterus remodeling and growth or whether they play a permissive role acting via different factors. Estrogens are known to influence the synthesis of growth factors such as epidermal growth factor (EGF) (Huet-Hudson et al. 1990) or insulin-like growth factor-I (Murphy et al. 1987) in the rat uterus. EGF receptor was shown to be regulated by androgens (Traish and Wotiz 1987) and this growth factor was shown to replace estrogen in respect to uterine and vaginal growth (Nelson et al. 1991). Growth factors are known to be important regulators in tissue remodeling. They are thought to act in the cross-talk of vascular cells such as endothelial cells, smooth muscle cells, blood born monocytes, and fibroblasts which are involved in vascular remodeling. Growth factors like EGF and TGFβ stimulate biosynthesis of extracellular matrix proteins, thus altering the composition and structure of the cellular environment.

9.5 Extracelullar Matrix and Cell Function

It is widely recognized that components of the extracellular matrix play an active role in regulating cell differentiation and function in embryological development, tissue repair, and disease (Rizzino 1988). Extracellular matrix proteins are involved in angiogenesis (Iruela-Arispe et al. 1991) and the differentiation of capillary endothelial cells (Kubota et al. 1988). Matrix components were also found to be actively involved in the release of cytokines from mononuclear cells (Pacifici et al. 1992). Further support for the involvement of extracellular matrix components in the transduction of hormone action are the findings that estrogen response on growth, morphological heterogeneity, and progesterone receptor induction was dependent on the cell substrate in cell culture (Pourreau-Schneider et al. 1984). It was shown that progestin receptor expression was enhanced in MCF-7 cells by estrogen treatment and this induction was augmented if cells were grown in a three-dimensional gel, as compared to growth as a monolayer.

Despite the fact that extracellular matrix proteins such as collagen and elastin show inherent self-assembly properties, cell phenotype will ultimately dictate composition and assembly of the extracellular matrix. The matrix in turn will influence motility, migration gene expression and growth. These effects are mediated by specific cellular receptors for matrix proteins, the integrins. These transmembrane glycoprotein receptors (reviewed by MacDonald 1989) are the transmembrane links between the extracellular matrix and the cytoskeleton (Burridge and Fath 1989). Thus changes in the composition of the extracellular matrix, e.g., induction of collagenases by estrogens (Too et al. 1986), will directly influence cell function via focal contact inbetween the altered extracellular matrix, its cellular receptors, and the cytoskeleton tightly bound to these receptors. In this respect, sexual dimorphism in hypertension and atherosclerosis may in part be explained by the modulating effect of sex steroids on extracellular matrix synthesis and degradation. This will ultimately lead to alteration in vascular remodeling and vascular responsiveness.

References

Berge LN, Hansen, J-B, Svensson B, Lyngmo V, Nordoy A (1990) Female Sex Hormones and Platelet/Endothelial interactions. Haemostasis 20:313-320

Brizzolara AL, Tomlinson A, Aberdeen J, Gourdie RG, Burnstock G (1992) Sex and Age as Factors Influencing the Vascular Reactivity in Watanabe Heritable Hyperlipidaemic Rabbits: A Pharmacological and Morphological Study of the Hepatic Artery. J Cardiovasc Pharmacol 19:86-95

Burridge K, Fath K (1989) Focal Contacts: Transmembrane Links between the Extracellular Matrix and the Cytoskeleton. Bio Essays 10:104-108

deSimone G, Deveraux RB, Roman MJ, Ganau A, Chien S, Alderman MH, Atlas St, Laragh JH (1991) Gender Differences in Left Ventricular Anatomy, Blood Viscosity and Volume Regulatory Hormones in Normal adults. Am J Cardiol 68:1704-1708

Huet-Hudson YM, Chakraborty C, De SK, Suzuki Y, Andrews GK, Dey SK (1990) Estrogen Regulates the Synthesis of Epidermal Growth Factor in Mouse Uterine Epithelial Cells. Mol Endocrinol 4:510-523

Iruela-Arispe ML, Diglio CA, Sage EH (1991) Modulation of Extracellular Matrix Proteins by Endothelial Cells Undergoing Angiogenesis In Vitro. Arteriosclerosis and Thrombosis 11:805-815

Kubota Y, Kleinmann HK, Martin GR, Lawley TJ (1988) Role of Laminin and Basement Membrane in the Morphological Differentiation of Human Endothelial Cells into Capillary-like Structures. J Cell Biol 107:1589-1598

Lin AL, Shain SA (1986) Sexual Dimorphism Characterizes Steroid Hormone Modulation of Rat Aortic Steroid Hormone Receptors. Endocrinology 119:296-302

Lobo RA (1990) Estrogens and Cardiovascular Disease. Ann NY Acad Sci 592:286-294

McDonald JA (1989) Receptors for Extracellular Matrix Components. Am J Physiol 257:L331-L337

Mitchell JRA, Schwartz CJ, Zinger A (1964) Relationship Between Aortic Plaques and Age, Sex, and Blood Pressure. Brit Med J 1:205-209

Murphy LJ, Murphy LC, Freisen HG (1987) Estrogen Induces Insulin-like Growth Factor-I in the Rat Uterus. Mol Endocrinol 1:445-450

Nelson KG, Takahashi T, Bossert NL, Walmer DK (1991) Epidermal Growth Factor Replaces Estrogen in the Stimulation of Female Genital-tract Growth and Differentiation. Proc Natl Acad Sci 88:21-25

Pacifici R, Basilico C, Roman J, Zutter MM, Santoro SA, McCracken R (1992) Collagen-induced Release of Interleukin 1 from Human Blood Mononuclear Cells. J Clin Invest 89:61.67

Pastore GN, DiCola LP, Dollahon NR, Gardner RM (1989) The Effect of Estradiol on Collagen Structure and Organization in the Immature Rat Uterus. PSEBM 191:69-77

Perrot-Applanat M, Groyer-Picard MT, Garcia E, Lorenzo F, Milgrom E (1988) Immunochemical Demonstration of Estrogen and Progesterone Receptors in Muscle Cells of Uterine Arteries in Rabbits and Humans. Endocrinology 123:1511-1519

Pommerantz K, Maddox Y, Maggi F, Ramey E, Ramwell PW (1980) Sex and Hormonal Modification of 6-keto-PGF_{1a} Release by Rat Aorta. Life Sciences 27:1233-1236

Pourreau-Schneider N, Berthois Y, Charpin MC, Jacquemier J (1984) Estrogen Response of MCF-7 Cells Grown on Diverse Substrates and in Suspension Culture: Promotion of Morphological Heterogeneity, Modulation of Progestin Receptor Induction; Cell-Substrate Interactions on Collagen Gels. J Steroid Biochem 21:763-771

Rajabi MR, Dodge GR, Solomon S, Poole AR (1991) Immunochemical and Immunohistological Evidence of Estrogen-Mediated Collagenolysis as a Mechanism of Cervical Dilatation in the Guinea Pig at Parturition. Endocrinology 128:371-378

Rhee CY, Spaet TH, Gaynor E, Lajan F, Shiang HH, Caruso E, Litwack RW (1974) Suppression of surgically induced vascular intimal hyperthrophy by estrogen. Circulation 49 (Suppl. III):III-9 (abstract)

Rizzino A (1988) Transforming Growth Factor-β: Multiple Effects on Cell Differentiation and Extracellular Matrices. Dev Biol 130:411-422

Stampfer MJ, Colditz GA, Willett WC, Manso JE, Rosner B, Speizer FE, Hennekens CH (1991) Postmenopausal Estrogen Therapy and Cardiovascular Disease. N Engl J Med 325:736-762

Too CKL, Kong JK, Greenwood, FC, Bryant-Greenwood GD (1986) The Effect of Oestrogen and Relaxin on Uterine and Cervical Enzymes: Collagenase, Proteoglycanase and β-Glucuronidase. Acta Endocrinol 111:394-403

Traish, AM, Wotiz HH (1987) Prostatic Epidermal Growth Factor Receptors and Their Regulation by Androgens. Endocrinology 121:1461-1467

Weidner G, Connor SL, Chesney MA, Burns JWE, Connor WE, Matarazzo JD, Mendell NR (1991) Sex Differences in High Density Lipoprotein Cholesterol Among Low-Level Alcohol Consumers. Circulation 83:176-180

Williams JK, Adams MR, Klopfenstein, HS (1990) Estrogen Modulates Responses of Atherosclerotic Coronary Arteries. Circulation 81:1680-1687

Wilson PWF, Garrison RJ, Castelli WP (1985) Postmenopausal estrogen use, cigarette smoking, and the cardiovascular morbidity in women over 50: the Framingham Study. N Engl J Med 313:1044-1049

Zhang A, Altura BT, Altura BM (1992) Endothelial-Dependent Sexual Dimorphism in Vascular Smooth Muscle: Role of Mg^{2+} and Na^+. Br J Pharmacol 105:305-310

10 Vascular Non-genomic Effects of Estrogen

Michel Farhat, Sylvie Abi-Younes, Roberto Vargas,
Raymond M. Wolfe, Robert Clarke, and Peter W. Ramwell

10.1 Introduction

Studies of the cellular mechanisms of action of steroids lead to extensive investigation of DNA-binding and gene regulatory proteins. Steroids are thought to passively diffuse into the cell and bind to their nuclear receptor protein. Each receptor is both ligand and cell specific, and binds to its respective steroid with high affinity (K_d: 0.1-1.0 nM). The ligand-receptor complex becomes an activated transcription factor, which binds gene regulatory elements on DNA to enhance transcription of several target genes. Protein synthesis and processing follows (Moudgil 1987).

Although many genes appear to require a few hours before alterations in their expression can be detected, some responses occur rapidly following administration of steroids. These "early responding genes" can be expressed within minutes of administration of the steroid (Landers and Spelsberg 1992). For example, the c-*myc* proto-oncogene mRNA in avian oviduct is decreased within 5 min of progesterone administration (Fink et al. 1988). An increase in transcription of the c-*myc* (Dubik et al. 1987) and *pS2* gene (Brown et al. 1984) in MCF-7 human breast cancer cells and the N-*myc* in rat uterus (Murphy et al. 1987) was observed within 15 min following estrogen administration. Estrogen also rapidly (5 min) inhibits c-*jun* gene expression in avian oviduct (Lau et al. 1990).

Although changes in mRNA expression may be detected within minutes, the functions mediated by these genes may not be altered until the appropriate mRNA has been translated and processed into mature protein. Estrogen can induce a two- to threefold increase in cAMP levels in rat uterus within 30 s (Szego and Davis 1969). These events that may be too rapid to involve genomic functions have therefore been designated "non-genomic" events (Duval et al. 1983; McEwen 1991). We propose to briefly review the literature on rapid steroid events, focusing on the vascular effects of estrogen. Where possible, we will relate the events to (a) steroid specificity, (b) reversibility, (c) absence of protein synthesis and (d) potency. Since few comprehensive studies have been published, the data reviewed will be fragmentary, but they will help to indicate what conditions need to be met for a definitive and convincing study. We will also describe some of our experiments in this area.

10.2 Steroids and Plasma Membranes

Steroids may bind to plasma membranes, inducing rapid cellular responses within seconds to minutes. Recently, Lan et al. (1990) reported that progesterone metabolites enhance the inhibitory effect of the mammalian GABA$_A$ receptor by interacting with the Cl$^-$ channel component of the GABA receptor complex. The progestin's interaction with the receptor complex opens the Cl$^-$ channel, leading to influx of Cl$^-$ into the neuron, making it less excitable. Progesterone also interacts with a membrane receptor to affect the maturation of *Xenopus* oocyte (Sadler and Maller 1982) and human sperm (Blackmore et al. 1990) by mobilizing extracellular Ca^{2+}.

The hypnotic and anesthetic properties of progestational steroids have been known for some time (Gyermek and Soyka 1968). Binding studies on synaptic (P2) membranes from brains of the amphibian *Taricha granulosa* indicate specific and high affinity (K_d: 0.5 nM) binding of radiolabeled corticosterone. The corticosterone membrane recognition site did not reveal any pharmacological similarity to the intracellular corticoid receptor (Orchinik et al. 1991). Similarly, glucocorticoid receptors were found to be randomly distributed on the cell membrane of S-49 lymphoma cells and are believed to mediate the cytolytic effect of glucocorticoids on lymphoid cell lines (Gametchu et al. 1991).

There is also evidence of interaction of estrogen with membrane components leading to rapid changes in membrane structure. Distinct morphological changes in luminal endometrial cells, evident by scanning electron microscopy, were detected following intravenous administration of 17β-estradiol or diethylstilbestrol. The number of microvilli was significantly increased within seconds and showed a dramatic regression 15-30 min following estrogen administration (Rambo and Szego 1983). In the central nervous system estrogen, like progesterone, influences neural activity and induces alterations in the electrical properties of neurons within minutes or seconds of application of the hormone (McEwen 1991). Microphoretic application of 17β-estradiol hemisuccinate induces a direct and immediate increase in firing frequency of the rat medial preoptic septal neurons in female rats (Kelly et al. 1977). Similarly, hippocampal slices from male rats show increased excitability of pyramidal cells after 10 min of 17β-estradiol application (Teyler et al. 1980). 17β-estradiol (10-100 nM) can also induce brief hyperpolarization and increased K^+ conductance in neurons of rat medial amygdala, even after suppression of protein synthesis (Nabekura et al. 1989). Furthermore, in the prolactin-secreting pituitary cell line, GH$_3$/B$_6$, 17β-estradiol (0.1-1 nM) was reported to generate an action potential within one minute of its application, and this effect was suppressed by Ca^{2+} channel blockade (Dufy et al. 1979).

10.3 Identification of Membrane Estrogen Receptors

Stereospecific hormone-membrane interactions which occur with high affinity indicate the presence of highly specific membrane binding sites for estrogen in various tissues, with K_d values ranging between 10 mM and 10 pM (Table 1). The isolation of purified membrane fractions for binding studies is of course controversial; membrane fractionation involves cell disruption, which obviously deranges the highly dynamic molecular events involved in hormone-membrane interaction. This may lead to aberrant redistribution of cytoplasmic and membrane constituents.

The occurrence of membrane associated binding sites has been claimed by use of affinity cytochemistry, classical receptor/ligand binding assays, and employment of large conjugated estrogen molecules that bind to cell membranes without altering the structural and functional integrity of the cell (Pietras and Szego 1977; Nenci et al. 1981; Nelson et al. 1986; Berthois et al. 1986). Many of these studies indicate a high degree of specificity, in that membrane binding of 17β-estradiol is unaffected by its 17α isomer, and that membrane estrogen binding sites are predominantly localized in cells known to be targets for estrogen action (Pietras and Szego 1979). Furthermore, warming produces a topographical rearrangement of estrogen binding to cell

Table 1. Identification of membrane binding sites for estrogen in various target tissues using different binding techniques

Binding method	Tissue	K_d (M)	References
Membrane fractions	Endometrium	10^{-3}	Pietras and Szego (1979)
	Brain	10^{-8}	Towle and Sze (1983)
	Liver	10^{-9}	Pietras and Szego(1980)
	Pituitary	10^{-11}	Bression et al. (1986)
		10^{-10}	Nenci et al. (1981)
	Breast cancer cells	-	Zanker et al. (1980)
Derivatized estrogen conjugates	Endometrium	-	Pietras and Szego (1977)
	Liver	10^{-9}	Pietras and Szego (1979)
Fluorescent estrogen conjugates	Breast cancer cells	10^{-8}	Nenci et al.(1981) Berthois et al. (1986)

surface with a pattern suggestive of estrogen binding to membrane proteins (Nenci et al. 1981).

10.4 Function of Membrane Estrogen Binding Sites

The nature of membrane estrogen binding sites and their relation to nuclear estrogen receptors remains obscure. Such binding sites may represent bona fide estrogen receptors, being products of the estrogen receptor gene. It is not clear how these receptors would mediate the non-genomic effects of steroids. Sequence analysis of steroid hormone receptors reveals a series of proteins with highly conserved structures. Steroid hormone receptors have five distinct domains (Green et al. 1986). However, none of these regions appear to possess recognizable signal transduction activities, other than those required to mediate transcriptional regulation within the nucleus. Although mutant estrogen receptors have been described, these are the result of alterations in the estrogen receptor gene (Fuqua et al. 1991). The presence of currently unidentified estradiol binding sites analogous to the corticosteroid membrane recognition site (Orchinik et al. 1991) cannot be excluded. These sites could represent novel membrane protein receptors, or highly specific "hydrophilic pockets" within the plasma membrane. Membrane steroid binding sites may be functional as receptors, inducing ion channeling and expression of intracellular second messengers.

Steroids could also alter membrane function without binding to a specific receptor-like protein. Cellular bilipid membranes contain both integrally and peripherally associated proteins incorporated into their fluid mosaic structure. Many of these membrane proteins are either chemically or structurally dependent upon their lipid environment in order to maintain their functionality (Lenaz et al. 1978). Steroid hormones are highly lipophilic and should partition predominantly into specific hydrophobic domains in the cell membrane. The cyclopentano moeities would be inserted into lipid, the more hydrophilic regions associating with more polar groups in the vicinity (Wilmer 1961). Thus, the C17 hydroxyl moeity of 17β-estradiol would be preferentially located within hydrophobic domains of the plasma membrane. The orientation of the C17-OH group confers stereospecificity on estradiol and could also confer the functional stereospecificity observed in some membrane-dependent responses.

Indirect local effects could also occur as a result of the insertion of steroids into specific "hydrophilic pockets" in the plasma membrane. 17β-estradiol can significantly reduce the fluidity of cellular membranes (Clarke et al. 1990). It has been suggested that the ability of estrogens to reduce the intracellular steady-state levels of both folate (Eilam et al. 1982) and methotrexate (Clarke et al. 1985) may reflect an estrogen-induced reduction in the fluidity of the cellular membrane. Perturbations in the folate membrane transport protein's local environment could inhibit function by altering the protein's conformation or decreasing protein mobility in the cell membrane (Clarke et al. 1990).

10.5 Rapid Estrogen-Mediated Events of Blood Vessels

Many of the components of the cardiovascular system, like the heart and organs that indirectly regulate cardiovascular function such as kidney, liver, adrenal, and pituitary, show nuclear accumulation and retention of estrogen (Stumpf 1990). Most of the cardiovascular effects of estrogen have been attributed to a regulatory genomic mechanism involving transcriptional events and acting at various levels of organization. However, estrogen may exert short-term effects on vascular tone via a direct effect on membrane electrical properties and ionic permeability.

Estradiol has a stereospecific effect on vascular reactivity of isolated arterial segments and perfused organ preparations. The contractile responses of isolated segments of the porcine left anterior descending coronary artery (LAD) and rat thoracic aorta segments to $PGF_{2\alpha}$ and phenylephrine, respectively, are inhibited after 5 min of incubation with 17β-estradiol (Vargas et al. 1989). 17α-estradiol, a weak estrogen, was a less potent inhibitor at the same concentration.

The inhibitory effect of 17β-estradiol is more pronounced in the coronary microcirculation. In the rat heart Langendorff preparation, a 5-min perfusion with 17β-estradiol (10 nM) elicits a dose-dependent inhibition of the norepinephrine-induced increase in perfusion pressure (Fig. 1). The greater sensitivity of the microcirculation to the effects of estrogen is of interest and may be due to the greater muscular composi-

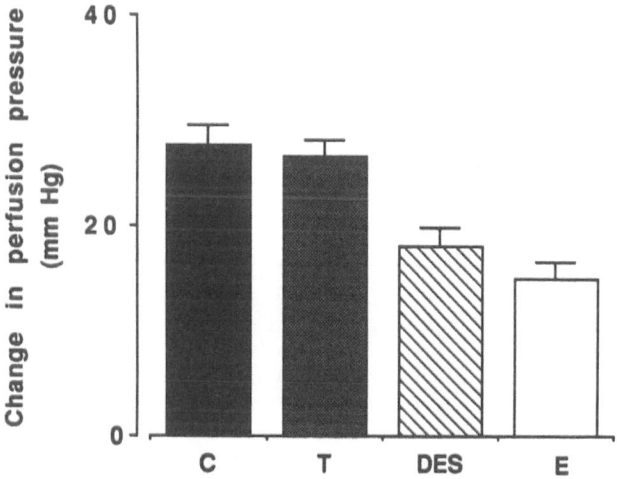

Fig. 1. Effect of 5 min perfusion with vehicle (*C*), or 100 n*M* concentrations of testosterone (*T*), diethylstilbestrol (*DES*) and 17β-estradiol (*E*) on NE-induced change in coronary perfusion pressure in the isolated rat heart preparation. Hearts were electrically paced at 300 bpm, and NE (32 μg) was administered as a bolus dose

tion of the vessels and/or to a greater abundance of estrogen receptors in the microvasculature.

There are qualitative differences in cardiovascular responses to estrogen. The effect of estrogen on the reactivity of two other vascular beds is different to that observed in the coronary circulation. In both pulmonary (Farhat and Ramwell 1992) and mesenteric (unpublished observation) beds, perfusion with nanomolar concentrations of 17β-estradiol elicits a significant potentiation of the pressor response to a number of agonists including norepinephrine, angiotensin II and the thromboxane mimic U46619. The effect is also observed with the non-steroidal estrogen diethylstilbestrol, but not with testosterone (Fig. 2). There is a high degree of specificity, since 17β-estradiol is more potent than its 17α isomer. The effect is also rapid and occurs in less than 5 min.

The mechanisms mediating the rapid effects of estradiol on vascular reactivity have not been identified. Since vascular reactivity in the

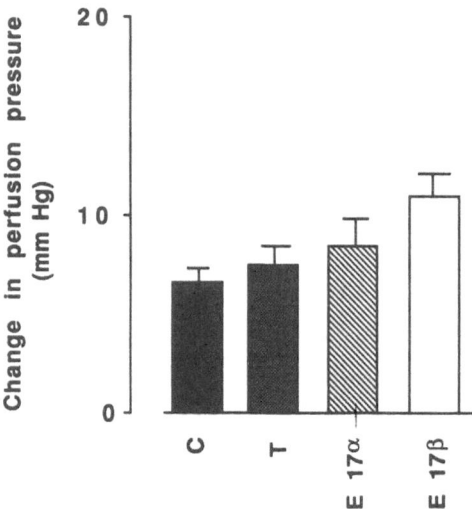

Fig. 2. Effect of 5 min perfusion with vehicle (*C*), or 10 n*M* concentrations of testosterone (*T*), estradiol 17α (*E 17α*) and 17β-estradiol (*E 17β*), on U46619-induced change in pulmonary perfusion pressure of the isolated rat lung. Lungs were perfused at a constant rate of 0.04 ml/g body weight, and U46619 (EC_{50}) infused via a side arm of the perfusion line

mesenteric circulation is predominantly regulated by the sympathetic nervous system, estrogen may exert its effect by potentiation of sympathetic neurotransmission (Iversen and Salt 1970) or regulation of adrenoceptor density (Williams and Lefkowitz 1977), and/or affinity (Colucci et al. 1982). However, the fact that the estrogenic effect is also observed with pressor agonists unrelated to adrenergic ligands suggests that estradiol may be acting on the contractile process.

Harder and Coulson (1979) found diethylstilbestrol to cause a dose-dependent membrane depolarization of vascular smooth muscle cells from dog coronary artery segments, by increasing K^+ conductance. Similar studies (De Beer and Keizer 1982) have shown a marked change in ionic permeability of the sarcolemma in rat atrial tissue, expressed as a change in the shape of the action potential. Low doses of 17β-estradiol (200 pg/ml) elicited an immediate and reversible shortening in the duration of the action potential. This effect was less pronounced in the presence of the Ca^{2+} channel blocker verapamil. Findings in accord with this observation were reported in rat aorta (Vargas et al. 1989), uterine artery (Stice et al. 1987), and in the isolated rabbit heart (Raddino et al. 1986), where the inhibitory effect of 17β-estradiol on the vascular pressor response was abolished in the absence of Ca^{2+}. All these observations suggest that the effect of estrogen on vascular reactivity may be mediated via a Ca^{2+}-dependent mechanism. The difference in the responses of the various vascular beds may be attributed to the large differences in Ca^{2+} kinetics (Van Breeman 1982).

10.6 Rapid Estrogen Effects on Cyclic Nucleotides

Estradiol may also have rapid effects on cyclic nucleotide turnover. Numano et al (1978) find that incubation of aortic segments from oophorectomized rabbits with 17α-estradiol (20 nM) for 5 min decreases both basal and epinephrine-stimulated cAMP levels. In contrast, uterine tissue from the same animals show increased cAMP levels under the same experimental conditions. These results are compatible with intravenous administration of 17β-estradiol (0.5 µg/100 g) to ovariectomized rats which also evokes a two- to threefold increase in uterine cAMP within 30 s (Szego and Davis 1969). Furthermore, activation of uterine adenylyl cyclase activity is also reported in castrated rats, 5 min after administration of the synthetic estrogen diethylstilbestrol (Rosenfeld and O'Malley 1970). We find that incubation of cultured pulmonary vascular smooth muscle cells treated with 17β-estradiol (0.1-10 µM) for 5 min exhibits a dose-dependent increase in cAMP levels. This effect is also observed with diethylstilbestrol but not with testosterone, nor is it affected by the protein synthesis inhibitor actinomycin D (unpublished observation). Thus, 17β-estradiol appears to increase cAMP levels by a rapid specific membrane effect, not related to genomic transcriptional events.

Estradiol may also rapidly inhibit guanylyl cyclase activity in vascular tissue. We have shown that in porcine left anterior descending coronary artery segments, 5-min incubation with 17β-estradiol (50 µM) inhibited both basal cGMP levels, as well as acetylcholine and sodium nitroprusside-stimulated levels (Fig. 3). The decrease in cGMP in this model correlated with an inhibitory effect of estrogen on both endothe-

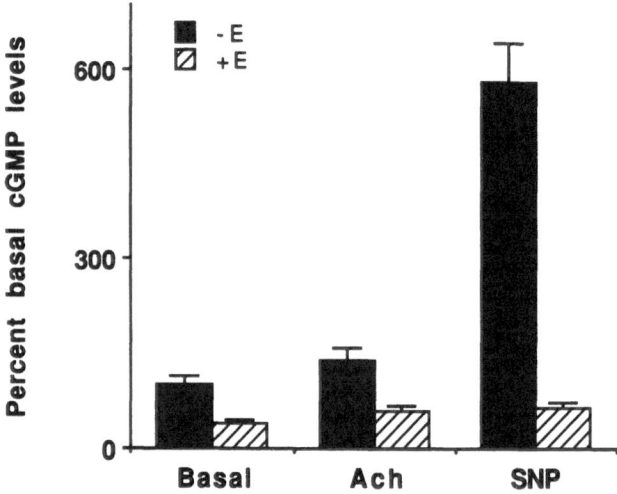

Fig. 3. Effect of 5 min incubation with 17β-estradiol (25 μM) on *basal* and acetylcholine- (*Ach*) and sodium nitroprusside (*SNP*)-stimulated cGMP levels in pig left anterior descending coronary artery

lium-dependent and endothelium-independent relaxations (Vargas et al. 1989). Similar inhibitory effects of 17β-estradiol on guanylyl cyclase activity were observed in isolated porcine internal mammary artery and in rat aortic segments (data not shown).

Estrogen may exert its effect on adenyl and guanylyl cyclases in three ways (Fig. 4): Firstly, by a direct action on the catalytic sites of the enzymes; secondly, by indirect activation of the regulatory G/F protein subunit (Sadler and Maller 1981). Bergamini et al. (1985) have shown, however, that stimulation of adenylate cyclase activity in endometrial membranes may occur in the absence of G protein activation, suggesting that the direct effect of estrogen on cyclase activity may be more important; thirdly, estrogen may increase cyclic nucleotide levels by indirectly regulating Ca^{2+} influx. One form of adenylate cyclase in the brain was found to be stimulated by Ca^{2+}-calmodulin interaction (Rosenberg and Storm 1987). Small amounts of calmodulin-sensitive cyclase have been identified in heart and lung tissue (Panchenko and Tkachuk 1984), but the relative importance of this

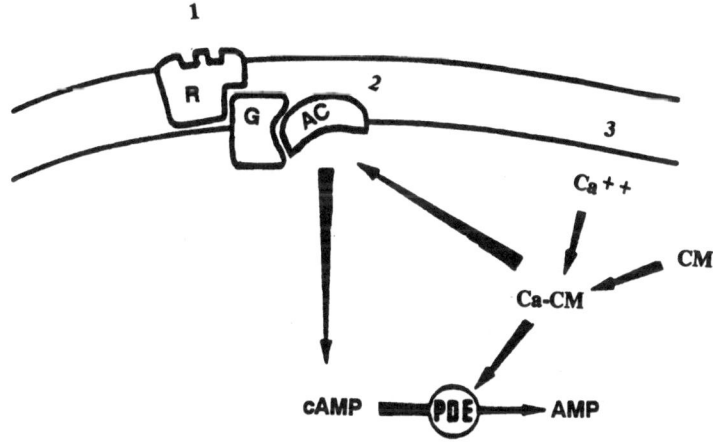

Fig. 4. The possible sites of action of estrogen on cyclic AMP turnover. *1*, Interaction with membrane estrogen receptor (*R*), and activation of regulatory proteins (*G*); *2*, direct stimulation of the catalytic site of the adenylyl cyclase enzyme (*AC*); *3*, regulation of intracellular Ca^{2+} levels, which interact with calmodulin (*CM*) and consequently activate AC or inhibit phosphodiesterase (*PDE*) activity

mechanism in the effects of estrogen is still unknown. Ca^{2+}-calmodulin interaction may also elevate cyclic nucleotide levels by inhibiting phosphodiesterase activity. Thus, one or more of these mechanisms may be involved in the effect of estradiol on cyclic nucleotide turnover in vascular tissue.

10.7 Conclusion

Rapid cardiovascular effects of 17β-estradiol and other potent estrogens are incompatible with the widely accepted steroidal genomic mechanism of action. The rapid nature of these responses may indicate a direct interaction with specific membrane binding sites or with specific membrane proteins. These interactions result in intracellular second messenger expression and ion fluxes. There is growing evidence to suggest "cross-talk" between membrane-associated receptors and intracellular steroid nuclear receptors. For example, Power et al. (1991) have shown that progesterone and estrogen receptors in transfected monkey kidney (CV1) cells can be activated by dopaminergic stimulation. This activation pathway was suggested to be a membrane receptor-mediated phosphorylation cascade, involving intracellular cAMP. Derivatives of cAMP have also been shown to substitute for progesterone and to mediate progesterone-dependent transcription in the absence of the hormone (Beyer et al. 1981; Denner et al. 1990).

The dose-response relationships and stereospecificity of membrane effects may provide some indication of the mechanism of action. Effects which occur predominantly at pharmacological concentrations ($\geq 1\mu M$) may be due to nonspecific effects or perturbations in membrane structure/function. At the lower physiological concentrations, we suggest that estrogens may promote ion flux and nucleotide synthesis through high affinity stereospecific cell membrane binding sites. The ion flux relates to changes in vascular smooth muscle tone, and it is possible that cyclic nucleotide synthesis may result in gene expression, as indicated by Power et al. (1991). The precise nature of these putative estrogen membrane binding sites remains to be elucidated.

Acknowledgments. This work was supported by NIHLBI grants HL36802 and HL40069

References

Bergamini C, Pansini F, Bettochi S Jr, Segala V, Dallochio F, Bagni B, Mollica G (1985) Hormonal sensitivity of adenylate cyclase from human endometrium: Modulation by estradiol. J Steroid Biochem 22(3): 299-303

Berthois Y, Pourreau-Schneider N, Gandilhon P, Mittre H, Tubiana N, Martin P (1986) Estradiol membrane binding sites on human breast cancer cell lines. Use of fluorescent estradiol conjugate to demonstrate plasma membrane binding systems. J Steroid Biochem 25:963-972

Beyer C, Canchola E, Larsson K (1981) Facilitation of lordosis behavior in the ovariectomized estrogen primed rat by dibutyryl cAMP. Physiol Behav 26: 249-251

Blackmore PF, Beebe SJ, Danforth DR, Alexander NA (1990) Progesterone and 17α-hydroxyprogesterone: Novel stimulators of calcium influx in human sperm. J Biol Chem 265: 1376-1380

Bression D, Michard M, Le Dafniet M, Pagesy P, Peillon F (1986) Evidence for a specific estradiol binding site on rat pituitary membranes. Endocrinology 119: 1048-1051

Brown A, Jeltsh J-M, Roberts M, Chambon P (1984) Activation of pS2 gene transcription is a primary response to estrogen in the human breast cancer cell line MCF-7. Proc Natl Acad Sci USA 81: 6344-6388

Clarke R, van den Berg HW, Kennedy DG, Murphy RF (1985) Estrogen receptor status and the response of human breast cancer cells to a combination of methotrexate and 17β-estradiol. Br J Cancer 51: 365-369

Clarke R, van den Berg HW, Murphy RF (1990) Tamoxifen and 17β-estradiol reduce the membrane fluidity of human breast cancer cells. J Natl Cancer Inst 82: 1702-1705

Colucci WS, Gimbrone M, McLaughlin MK, Halpern W, Alexander RW (1982) Increased vascular catecholamine sensitivity and alpha adrenergic receptor affinity in female and estrogen treated male rats. Circ Res 50: 805-811

De Beer E, Keizer H (1982) Direct action of estradiol 17β on the atrial action potential. Steroids 40: 223-231

Denner LA, Weigel NL, Maxwell BL, Schrader WT, O'Malley BW (1990) Regulation of progesterone receptor-mediated transcription by phosphorylation. Science 250: 1740-1743

Dubik D, Dembinski TC, Shiu RPC (1987) Stimulation of c-myc oncogene expression associated with estrogen-induced proliferation of human breast cancer cells. Cancer Res. 47: 6517-6521

Dufy B, Vincent JD, Fleury H, du Pasquier P, Gourdji D, Tixier-Vidal A (1979) Membrane effect of thyrotropin releasing hormone and estrogen shown by intracellular recording from pituitary cells. Science 204: 509-511

Farhat MY, Ramwell PW (1992) Estradiol potentiates the vasopressor response of the isolated perfused rat lung to the thromboxane mimic U46619. J Pharmacol Exp Ther (in press)

Fink KL, Wieben ED, Woloschak GE, Spelsberg TC (1988) Rapid regulation of c-myc proto-oncogene expression by progesterone in the avian oviduct. Proc Natl Acad Sci USA 85: 1796-1800

Fuqua SAW, Fitzgerald SD, Chamness GC, Tandon AK, McDonnel DP, Nawaz Z, O'Malley BW, McGuire WL (1991) Variant human breast tumor estrogen receptor with constitutive transcriptional activity. Cancer Res 51: 105-109

Gametchu B, Watson CS, Pasko D (1991) Size and steroid binding characterization of membrane-associated glucocorticoid receptor in S-49 lymphoma cells. Steroids 56:402-419

Green S, Walter P, Kumar V, Krust A, Bornert J-M, Argos P, Chambon P (1986) Human oestrogen receptor cDNA: sequence, expression and homology to v-erb-A. Nature 320: 134-139

Gyermek L, Soyka LF (1975) Steroid anesthetics. Anesthesiology 42:331-344

Ham E, Zanetti M, Goldberg N, Kuehl F Jr (1974) Alterations in uterine cGMP levels in the cycling rat. Fed Proc 33:268

Harder D, Coulson P (1979) Estrogen receptors and effects of estrogen on membrane electrical properties of coronary vascular smooth muscle. J Cell Physiol 100: 375-382

Iversen LL, Salt PJ (1970) Inhibition of catecholamine uptake-2 by steroids in the isolated rat heart. Br J Pharmacol 40: 528-530

Kelly R, Abel M (1980) Catecholestrogens stimulate and direct prostaglandin synthesis. Prostaglandins 20: 613-626

Lan NC, Chen J-S, Belelli D, Pritchett DB, Seeburg PH, Gee KW (1990) A steroid recognition site is functionally coupled to an expressed GABA benzodiazepine receptor. Eur J Pharmacol 188: 403-406

Landers JP, Spelsberg TC (1992) New concepts in steroid hormone action: Transcription factors, proto-oncogenes, and the cascade model for steroid regulation of gene expression. Critic Rev Eukar Gene Express 2: 19-63

Lau CK, Subramaniam M, Rasmussen K, Spelsberg TC (1990) Rapid inhibition of the c-jun proto-oncogene expression in avian oviduct by estrogen. Endocrinology 127: 2595-2597

Lenaz G, Curatola G, Mazzanti L, Parenti-Castelli G (1978) Biophysical studies on agents affecting the state of membrane lipids: Biochemical and pharmacological implications. Mol Cell Biochem 22: 3-32

McEwen B (1991) Non-genomic and genomic effects of steroids on neural activity. TIPS 12:141-147

Moudgil VK, ed. Recent advances in steroid hormone action. Walter de Gruyter, New York, 1987

Murphy LJ, Murphy LC, Friesen HG (1987) Estrogen induction of n-myc and c-myc proto-oncogene expression in the rat uterus. Endocrinology 120: 1882-1888

Nabekura J, Oomura Y, Minani T, Mizuno Y, Fukuda A (1986) Mechanisms of the rapid effect of 17β-estradiol on medial amygdala neurons. Science 223: 226-228

Nenci I, Marchetti E, Marzola A (1981) Affinity cytochemistry visualizes specific estrogen binding sites on the plasma membrane of breast cancer cells. J Steroid Biochem 14: 1139-1146

Numano F (1978) In vitro effects of estrogen on cyclic nucleotides in the arterial wall. In: Hauss et al. eds International symposium: State of prevention and therapy in human arteriosclerosis and in animal models. 373-383

Orchinik M, Murray TF, Moore FL (1991) A corticosteroid receptor in neuronal membranes. Science 252: 1848-1851

Panchenko MP, Tkachuck VA (1984) Calmodullin activates adenylate cyclase from rabbit heart plasma membranes. FEBS Lett 174: 50-54

Pietras R, Szego C (1977) Specific binding sites for oestrogen at the outer surface of isolated endometrial cells. Nature 265: 69-72

Pietras R, Szego C (1979) Metabolic and proliferative responses to estrogen by hepatocytes selected for plasma membrane binding sites for estradiol-17β. J Cell Physiol 98: 145-160

Pietras R, Szego C (1980) Partial purification and characterization of oestrogen receptors in subfractions of hepatocyte plasma membranes. Biochem J 191: 743-760

Power RF, Mani S, Codina J, Conneely OM, O'Malley BW (1991) Dopaminergic and ligand-independent activation of steroid hormone receptors. Science 254: 1636-1639

Raddino R, Manca C, Poli E, Bolognesi R, Visioli O (1986) Effects of 17β estradiol on the isolated rabbit heart. Arch Int Pharmacodyn 281: 57-65

Rambo C, Szego C (1983) Estrogen action at endometrial membranes: Alterations in luminal surface detectable within seconds. J Cell Biol 97: 679-685

Rosenberg GB, Storm DR (1987) Immunological distinction between calmodulin-sensitive and calmodulin-insensitive adenylate cyclases. J Biol Chem 16: 7623-7628

Rosenfeld M, O'Malley B (1970) Steroid hormones: Effects on adenyl cyclase activity and adenosine 3', 5' monophosphate in target tissues. Science 168: 253-255

Sadler SE, Maller JL (1981) Progesterone inhibits adenylate cyclase in Xenopus oocytes. Action on the guanine nucleotide regulatory protein. J Biol Chem 256: 6368-6373

Sadler SE, Maller JL (1982) Identification of a steroid receptor on the surface of Xenopus oocytes by photoaffinity labeling. J Biol Chem 257: 355-361

Stice S, Ford S, Rosazza J, Van Orden D (1987) Role of 4-hydroxylated estradiol in reducing Ca^{2+} uptake of uterine smooth muscle cells through potential sensitive channels. Biol Reprod 36: 361-368

Stumpf WE (1990) Steroid hormones and the cardiovascular system: Direct actions of estradiol, progesterone, testosterone, gluco- and mineralocorticoids, and soltriol (vitamin D) on central nervous regulatory and peripheral tissues. Experientia 46: 13-25

Szego C, Davis J (1969) Inhibition of estrogen-induced cyclic AMP elevation in rat uterus by glucocorticoids. Life Sc 8: 1109-1116

Teyler T, Vardaris R, Lewis D, Rawitch A (1980) Gonadal steroids: Effects on excitability of hippocampal pyramidal cells. Science 209: 1017-1019

Towle A, Sze P (1983) Steroid binding to synaptic plasma membrane: Differential binding of glucocorticoids and gonadal steroids. J Steroid Biochem 18: 135-143

Van Breeman C, Mangel A, Fahim M, Meisheri K (1982) Selectivity of calcium antagonistic action in vascular smooth muscle. Am J Cardiol 49: 507-510

Vargas R, Thomas G, Wroblewska B, Ramwell PW (1989) Differential effects of 17α and 17β-estradiol on PGF2α mediated contraction of the porcine coronary artery. Adv Prost Thromb Leuk Res 19: 277-280

Williams LT, Lefkowitz RJ (1977) Regulation of rabbit myometrial alpha adrenergic receptors by estrogen and progesterone. J Clin Invest 60:815-818

Zanker K, Prokscha G, Blumel G (1980) Plasma membrane integrated estrogen receptors in breast tissue: Possible modulation molecules for intracellular hormone level. Eur J Cancer Clin Oncol 100: 135-148

11 Effects of Estrogens and Progestins on Atherosclerosis in Primates

Michael R. Adams, Janice D. Wagner, and Thomas B. Clarkson

11.1 Effects of Estrogen Deficiency and Hormone Replacement

In human populations where coronary heart disease is a major public health problem, the incidence of coronary heart disease is much lower in premenopausal women than in men of similar age. This gender difference is paralleled by a difference in extent and severity of coronary artery atherosclerosis (McGill and Stern 1979). It is widely believed that ovarian estrogen is responsible for this relative sparing of the coronary arteries; however, it remains uncertain whether risk of coronary heart disease or atherosclerosis in human beings is influenced by conditions (e.g., menopause, pregnancy) that affect endogenous estrogen concentrations (Adams et al. 1987). Although, there is compelling evidence that estrogen replacement therapy results in a marked reduction in risk of coronary heart disease in postmenopausal women (Bush 1990), the mechanisms by which this effect is mediated are poorly understood. Among multiple possibilities are inhibitory effects on atherosclerosis progression, or coronary thrombosis and beneficial effects on vasomotor function of coronary arteries. We summarize here the experimental evidence regarding effects of estrogen deficiency and hormone replacement therapy on coronary artery atherosclerosis.

This discussion emphasizes coronary arteries because: (1) The gender difference in atherosclerosis extent is confined to coronary arteries (McGill and Stern 1979); (2) experimental evidence indicates that effects of sex hormones are confined to coronary arteries and, perhaps, femoral arteries (McGill and Stern 1979; Adams et al. 1987; Clarkson et al. 1990); and (3) effects on coronary arteries are of greatest relevance to coronary heart disease, the major clinical sequela of atherosclerosis in human beings. Effects on aortic atherosclerosis, for example, may be of limited relevance and, in fact, may lead to inappropriate conclusions regarding coronary heart disease.

Some of the initial pieces of evidence that estrogen inhibits the progression of coronary artery atherosclerosis emerged from a series of studies done in the 1950s at the Michael Reese Research Institute. Among the important findings from these studies was that hens were resistant to development of coronary artery atherosclerosis relative to roosters (Stamler et al. 1954). Furthermore, ligation of the hen oviduct, which results in a marked elevation in plasma cholesterol concentration, had no effect on the relative resistance of the hen to atherosclerosis, while ovariectomy resulted in a marked exacerbation of atherosclerosis (Stamler et al. 1954). In addition, exogenous estradiol in physiologic doses was found to inhibit progression of atherosclerosis (Pick et al. 1952) and to promote regression of atherosclerosis (Pick et al. 1952) in this species. Subsequent studies using White Carneau pigeons resulted in similar conclusions regarding inhibitory effects of physiologic doses of estrogen on coronary atherosclerosis (Prichard et al. 1966).

The subject of sex hormones and atherosclerosis received relatively little attention in the 1960s and 1970s. In 1977, McGill and colleagues studied the effects of endogenous estrogens on atherosclerosis extent in ovariectomized baboons. These investigators determined that ovariectomy was not associated with increased extent or severity of diet-induced atherosclerosis. Furthermore, there were no significant effects of treatment with either physiologic or pharmacologic estrogen replacement therapy. It is perhaps important to note that, unlike many other primate species (including man), the baboon is relatively resistant to diet-induced hyperlipidemia and atherosclerosis. Furthermore, there is no gender difference in the extent of diet-induced coronary artery atherosclerosis in the baboon.

In our laboratory, we have utilized the cynomolgus macaque (*Macaca fascicularis*) to study effects of reproductive steroids on coronary artery atherosclerosis. This nonhuman primate species has been used in atherosclerosis research for approximately 30 years, principally because of its susceptibility to diet-induced atherosclerotic involvement of main branch coronary arteries. We chose it for our research because, in addition to its susceptibility to atherosclerosis, its reproductive physiology is very similar to that of human beings; the female has a 30-day menstrual cycle and circulating sex hormone patterns which are similar to those of women (Adams et al. 1985) and a natural menopause occurs in aged monkeys.

In an initial study of the relationship between endogenous sex steroids and atherosclerosis, cynomolgus macaques were fed a moderately atherogenic diet containing 40% of calories as fat and 0.4 mg of cholesterol per calorie. There were four experimental groups: males ($n = 15$), intact nonpregnant females ($n = 23$), surgically postmenopausal (i.e., ovariectomized) females ($n = 21$), and pregnant females ($n = 27$). Total plasma cholesterol, plasma high density lipoprotein (HDL) cholesterol concentrations and blood pressure were determined periodically. After 30 months, all animals were necropsied and the extent of atherosclerosis (lesion cross-sectional area) was determined morphometrically.

The results are summarized in Fig. 1. As in a previous study (Hamm et al. 1983), males were found to have more extensive coronary artery atherosclerosis relative to intact nonpregnant females (Kaplan et al. 1984). Males also had significantly lower plasma HDL-cholesterol concentrations and higher systolic blood pressure. Ovariectomy (i.e., estrogen deficiency) resulted in a more atherogenic plasma lipoprotein pattern (decreased plasma HDL-cholesterol and increased total plasma cholesterol concentrations), and a twofold increase in coronary artery atherosclerosis extent (Adams et al. 1985). The hyperestrogenic state of pregnancy was associated with a marked reduction in extent of coronary artery atherosclerosis (Adams et al. 1987). In this group of animals, both total plasma cholesterol and HDL- cholesterol concentrations were markedly decreased during pregnancy.

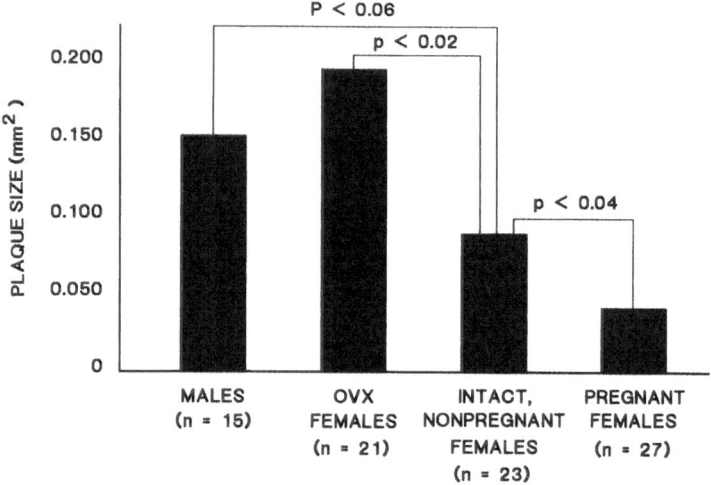

Fig. 1. Extent of diet-induced coronary artery atherosclerosis (plaque size) in cynomolgus monkey males, intact females, ovariectomized females and pregnant females

The results of this study provide indirect evidence regarding the effects of endogenous sex hormones on atherosclerosis extent. Males and ovariectomized females do not differ in regard to coronary artery atherosclerosis extent and also have consistently low plasma estradiol concentrations in the range of 20 pg/ml. Atherosclerosis extent is reduced by approximately one half in intact, nonpregnant females, which have much higher plasma estradiol concentrations (normal range of 60-300 pg/ml depending on time of the menstrual cycle). Atherosclerosis extent is reduced by approximately one fourth in pregnant females, animals which experienced sustained dramatic elevations in plasma estradiol concentrations (300-1000 pg/ml).

Direct evidence for an inhibitory effect of physiologic estrogen concentrations on progression of coronary artery atherosclerosis is provided by the results of a subsequent study (Adams et al. 1990). Ovariectomized monkeys were assigned randomly to one of three treatment groups: (1) no hormone replacement ($n = 17$); (2) continually administered 17β-estradiol plus cyclically administered progesterone ($n = 20$);

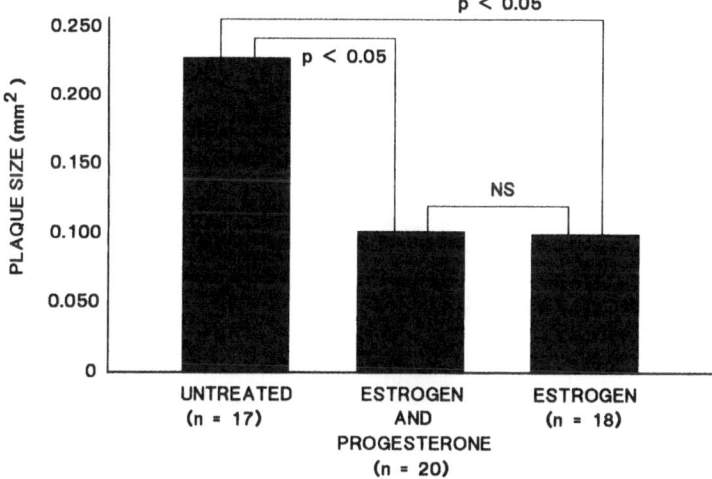

Fig. 2. Extent of diet-induced coronary artery atherosclerosis (plaque size) in ovariectomized monkeys receiving no hormone treatment, treatment with 17β-estradiol or 17β-estradiol plus progesterone

and (3) continuously administered 17β-estradiol ($n = 18$). Physiologic patterns of plasma estradiol and progesterone concentrations were maintained by administering the hormones in sustained-release subcutaneous Silastic implants. The experiment lasted 30 months. At necropsy, coronary artery atherosclerosis was reduced by approximately one half in animals in both hormone replacement groups (Fig. 2). Anti-atherogenic effects of hormone replacement were independent of variation in total plasma cholesterol, lipoprotein cholesterol, apoprotein A1 and B concentrations, average low density lipoprotein (LDL) particle size, and high density lipoprotein subfractional heterogeneity. Similarly, effects of hormone replacement on atherosclerosis could not be accounted for by other risk variables, i.e., blood pressure or carbohydrate tolerance. These finding suggest that an inhibitory influence of estrogen on atherogenesis and coronary heart disease must be mediated either through other risk factors not assessed in this study or through a direct influence on cellular or biochemical events occurring in the arterial intima.

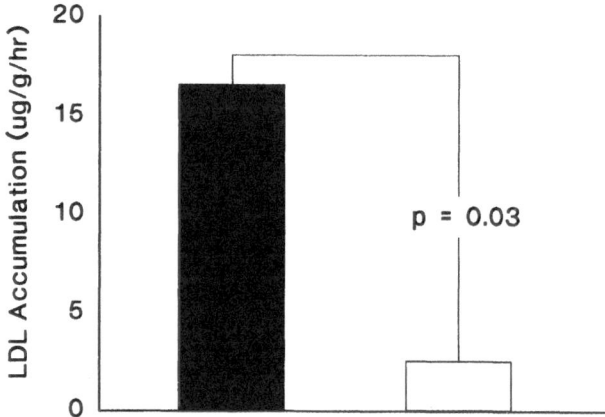

Fig. 3. Effect of estrogen replacement therapy on accumulation of LDL degradation products (µg/g artery/h) in ovariectomized monkeys. *Solid bar,* no
treatment; *open bar,* parenteral estradiol + progesterone (mg/dl)

To determine the mechanism that could account for the protective
effect of estradiol observed in our studies, we used radiolabeled LDL
coupled with tyramine cellobiose, a residualizing label, to measure intracellular accumulation of LDL and LDL degradation products in arteries of female cynomolgus monkeys (Wagner et al. 1991). We studied coronary arteries of surgically postmenopausal cynomolgus
monkeys fed an atherogenic diet and either treated or not treated with
parenterally administered 17β-estradiol and progesterone.

The accumulation of LDL degradation products was greatly diminished by estrogen replacement therapy (Fig. 3). This indicates a
mechanism by which estrogen may inhibit atherogenesis directly at the
level of the arterial intima, and may account for the unexplained variability in the effects of estrogens and progestins on atherosclerosis and
coronary heart disease risk.

11.2 Effects of Oral Contraceptives

Effects of combination oral contraceptives on CHD risk continue to be controversial (Mishell 1988). Although these compounds have been in widespread use for 25 years, there is no compelling evidence that there has been a widespread adverse influence on CHD risk. On the contrary, CHD incidence among women in the United States has declined markedly over the same period. Also, while there is a well-known increase in CHD risk associated with current oral contraceptive use, present evidence indicates that this increase is largely confined to users of older, high-dose contraceptive formulations who are also cigarette smokers (Mishell 1988; Realini and Goldzieher 1985; Throneycroft 1990; Thorogood and Vessey 1990). This increase in risk disappears after cessation of oral contraceptive use, suggesting that a nonatherogenic mechanism such as thrombosis or vasospasm is responsible. Furthermore, some studies have actually suggested a decreased risk in past users of oral contraceptives (Stampfer et al. 1990), while none provide compelling evidence for an increased CHD risk. Taken together, these epidemiologic findings indicate that oral contraceptives probably do not accelerate, and may in fact inhibit, progression of atherosclerosis. Further evidence to support this conclusion is provided by the work of Engel et al. (1983) who studied premenopausal women undergoing coronary angiography for the diagnosis of myocardial infarction. These investigators found that, in contrast with oral contraceptive nonusers, users had little or no angiographic evidence of coronary artery atherosclerosis.

Because of the great difficulty in studying the effects of oral contraceptives on pathogenesis of atherosclerosis in human beings, we have used the cynomolgus macaque model to examine this question.

In an initial experiment (Adams et al. 1987), we compared the effects of an oral contraceptive (ethinyl estradiol and norgestrel), an intravaginal ring (17β-estradiol and levonorgestrel), and a placebo vaginal ring (no hormone treatment). Animals consumed an atherogenic diet for a total of 31 months.

Neither contraceptive treatment influenced prevalence of atherosclerosis. However, treatment did influence extent of coronary artery atherosclerosis, i.e., plaque size. Treatment with the intravaginal ring resulted in plaques that were larger than those of both control females

Table 1. Plasma HDL cholesterol concentration and coronary artery atherosclerosis in contraceptive-treated and control monkeys

Groups	Plaque prevalence	Plaque area[a] (mm[b])	Plasma HDL[a] (mg/dl)
Untreated controls ($n = 15$)	9/15	0.549 ± 0.081	40 ± 5
Contraceptive vaginal ring ($n = 13$)	7/13	0.870 ± 0.138^2	25 ± 2^c
Oral contraceptive ($n = 15$)	6/15	0.470 ± 0.135	22 ± 2^c

[a]Mean $\pm$ SEM
[b]Different from control and oral contraceptive groups, $p < 0.05$
[c]Different from control group, $p < 0.01$

and oral contraceptive treated females (Table 1). This difference in atherosclerosis extent occurred despite the fact that plasma HDL cholesterol concentrations were reduced markedly and to the same extent in both contraceptive-treated groups. The result suggested that the much greater estrogenic influence associated with the ethinyl estradiol-containing oral contraceptive resulted in inhibition of atherosclerosis despite the pronounced progestin-induced lowering of plasma HDL concentrations. A subsequent study was designed to further clarify these relationships.

We compared oral contraceptives that contained equivalent amounts of ethinyl estradiol (50 µg) but structurally and pharmacologically different progestins, norgestrel (500 µg) and ethynodiol diacetate (1 mg) (Clarkson et al. 1990). Despite the expected marked influences on plasma lipoproteins, i.e., decreased plasma HDL-cholesterol concentrations and increased total plasma cholesterol to HDL-cholesterol ratio (Fig. 4), the extent of coronary artery atherosclerosis was decreased by both oral contraceptives. This effect was especially pronounced among females at highest risk due to "atherogenic" plasma lipid profiles (pretreatment total plasma cholesterol: HDL-cholesterol > 4.5) (Fig. 5).

As estimated by multiple regression analysis, there was a dramatic disparity between observed extent of coronary artery atherosclerosis

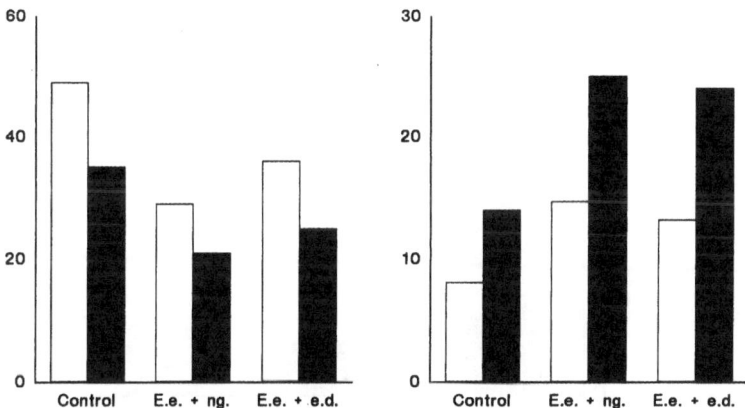

Fig. 4. Plasma high density lipoprotein (HDL) cholesterol concentration (*left panel*) and total plasma cholesterol to HDL cholesterol ratio (*right panel*) in *control* (no hormone treatment), ethinyl estradiol + norgestrel (*E.e. + ng.*)-treated and ethinyl estradiol + ethynodiol diacetate (*E.e. + e.d.*)-treated monkeys. Data are presented for all animals ($n = 71$; *open bars*) and for those at high risk (*solid bars*) of atherosclerosis due to pretreatment TPC to HDL cholesterol > 4.5 ($n = 32$). For effects of treatment, $p < 0.01$

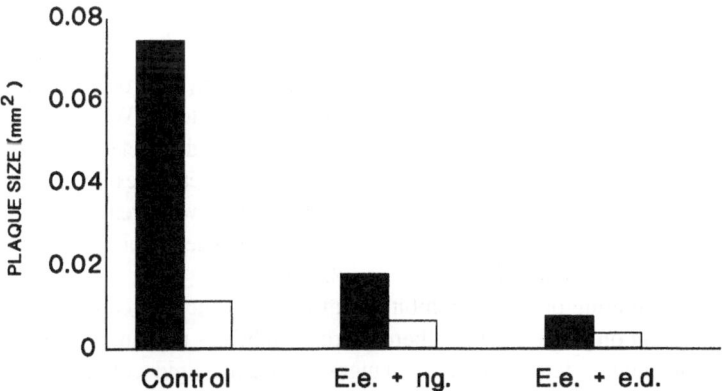

Fig. 5. Atherosclerotic plaque size in coronary arteries of *control* (no hormone treatement), ethinyl estradiol + norgestrel (*E.e. + ng.*)-treated and ethinyl estradiol + ethynodiol diacetate (*E.e. + e.d*)-treated monkeys. Data are presented for all animals ($n = 71$; *open bars*) ($p = 0.15$ for an effect of treatment) and for those at high risk (*solid bars*) due to pretreatment total plasma cholesterol to HDL cholesterol > 4.5 ($p = 0.02$ for an effect of treatment)

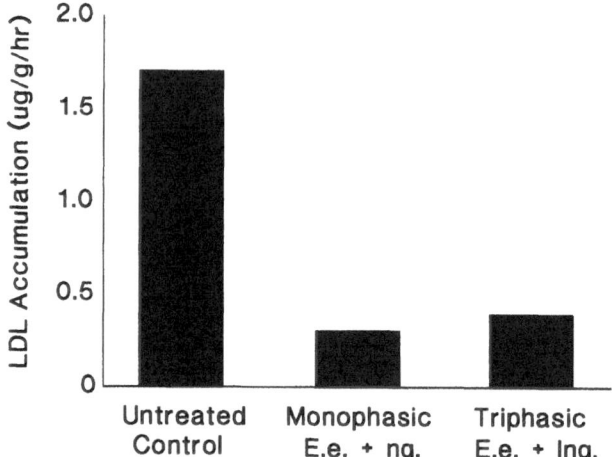

Fig. 6. Rate of accumulation of products of low density lipoprotein (*LDL*) degradation in coronary arteries of untreated monkeys, monkeys treated with a monophasic oral contraceptive containing ethinyl estradiol + norgestrel (*E.e.* + *ng.*) or a triphasic oral contraceptive containing ethinyl estradiol + levonorgestrel (*E.e.* + *lng.*). For effect of treatment, $p > 0.05$

and extent of atherosclerosis predicted by theoretically atherogenic effects of the oral contraceptives on plasma lipoprotein patterns. When all animals are considered, an approximate doubling of atherosclerosis extent was predicted, while a 50–75% reduction in atherosclerosis extent was observed. Among the high-risk individuals, the contrast was even more striking. A doubling of atherosclerosis was again predicted, while a 75–85% decrease in atherosclerosis extent was observed.

The finding of a large inhibitory influence of the oral contraceptive treatment on progression of atherosclerosis indicates that, in terms of atherogenicity, steroid-induced changes in plasma lipid concentrations are not the same as changes induced by diet. We have hypothesized that this atherosclerosis-inhibiting effect is due to the ethinyl estradiol component of the oral contraceptives.

In seeking the mechanism of the observed protective effect of ethinyl estradiol, we again used radiolabeled LDL coupled with tyramine cellobiose to measure intracellular accumulation of low density lipo-

protein (LDL) and LDL degradation products in arteries of female cynomolgus monkeys (Wagner et al. 1991). The animals were fed a
moderately atherogenic diet, either with or without oral contraceptive
treatment, for 16 weeks. The results of these studies are summarized in
Fig. 6. The oral contraceptives, a monophasic preparation containing
50 µg ethinyl estradiol and 500 µg norgestrel and a triphasic preparation containing 30-40 µg ethinyl estradiol and 50-125 µg levonorgestrel, both induced a more atherogenic lipid profile (decreased plasma
HDL-cholesterol, increased total plasma cholesterol: HDL-cholesterol)
compared to diet only, yet the accumulation of LDL degradation products in the coronary arteries was significantly reduced. This finding is
consistent with the data of Haarbo et al. (1991), who studied the effects
of exogenous estrogen and estrogen-progestin combinations on arterial
cholesterol accumulation in rabbits fed an atherogenic diet. In these
studies, arterial cholesterol accumulation was reduced by one third in
rabbits treated with 17β-estradiol, given either alone or in combination
with the contraceptive progestins norethindrone and levonorgestrel.
This effect was not explained by variation in plasma lipoproteins.

This finding suggests a mechanism by which oral contraceptives
may inhibit atherogenesis directly at the level of the arterial intima,
even in the face of marked reductions in plasma HDL-cholesterol concentrations.

11.3 Summary and Conclusions

We have used the cynomolgus macaque as a model for the study of the
effects of endogenous and exogenous sex steroid hormones on atherosclerosis. As in human beings, premenopausal female cynomolgus macaques develop much less extensive coronary artery atherosclerosis
than their male counterparts. Furthermore, surgical menopause results
in a more atherogenic plasma lipoprotein pattern and an approximate
doubling of atherosclerosis extent. Physiological replacement with
17β-estradiol alone or in combination with progesterone prevents the
increase in coronary artery atherosclerosis extent associated with ovariectomy. This effect is independent of plasma lipoprotein concentrations and appears to be accounted for, at least in part, by an inhibitory
effect of estrogen replacement therapy on the uptake and degradation

of LDL by the artery wall. Also, as in human beings, treatment with certain types of combination oral contraceptives results in a marked decrease in plasma HDL-cholesterol concentration. Nonetheless, coronary artery atherosclerosis extent is reduced in monkeys by this treatment, with the most pronounced effect among animals at highest risk due to theoretically adverse plasma lipoprotein profiles. As with estrogen replacement therapy, this effect can be accounted for, at least in part, by inhibition of the uptake and degradation of LDL by the artery wall.

The evidence from these studies suggests a mechanism by which antiatherogenic effects of both physiologic and pharmacologic concentrations of estrogen may be mediated. The accumulation of cholesterol is a central characteristic of the development of atherosclerotic plaque (Steinberg et al. 1989). Since plasma LDL is the major source of this cholesterol (Steinberg et al. 1989), factors that inhibit the uptake and degradation of LDL by the arterial wall can be assumed to result in inhibition of atherosclerosis.

It should be noted that other factors may also be involved. Estrogen and progesterone receptors have been found in arterial endothelial and smooth muscle cells of several species, including human beings (Ingegno et al. 1988; Lin et al. 1982; Lin et al. 1986). It has been shown that treatment of baboons with estrogen results in a redistribution of arterial intracellular estrogen receptors and an increase in the cellular concentration of progesterone receptors (Lin et al. 1986). These findings imply a role for sex steroids in the regulation of arterial cell function. Other animal studies have shown that estrogen treatment results in reductions in lipoprotein-induced arterial smooth muscle cell proliferation (Fischer-Dzoga et al. 1983), inhibition of the myointimal proliferation associated with mechanical endothelial injury (Rhee et al. 1974; Rhee et al. 1978; Weigensberg et al. 1984), reduced arterial cholesterol ester influx, hydrolysis and accumulation (Haarbo et al. 1991; Hough and Zilversmit 1986), inhibition of platelet aggregation (Johnson et al. 1977), decreased collagen and elastin production (Fischer 1972; Wolinsky 1972; Fischer and Swain 1977; Beldekas et al. 1981), and increased prostacyclin production by arterial smooth muscle cells (Chang et al. 1980). These studies indicate that estrogen may inhibit atherogenesis by inhibiting foam cell formation, platelet aggregation, smooth muscle cell proliferation, and the accumulation of collagen and elastin.

References

Adams MR, Clarkson TB, Kaplan JR, Koritnik DR (1985) Ovariectomy, social status, and coronary artery atherosclerosis in cynomolgus monkeys. Arteriosclerosis 5:192-200

Adams MR, Kaplan JR, Koritnik DR (1985) Psychosocial influences on ovarian endocrine and ovulatory function in cynomolgus monkeys (*Macaca fascicularis*). Physiol Behav 35:935-940

Adams MR, Clarkson TB, Koritnik DR, Nash HA (1987) Contraceptive steroids and coronary artery atherosclerosis in cynomolgus macaques. Fertil Steril 47:1010-1018

Adams MR, Kaplan JR, Clarkson TB, Koritnik DR (1987) Pregnancy-associated inhibition of coronary artery atherosclerosis in monkeys: evidence of a relationship with endogenous estrogen. Arteriosclerosis 7:378-384

Adams MR, Kaplan JR, Clarkson TB, Koritnik DR (1987) Effects of psychosocial stress, menopause and pregnancy on coronary artery atherosclerosis. In: Eaker ED, Packard B, Wenger NK, Clarkson TB, Tyroler HA (Eds.). Coronary Heart Disease in Women. Haymarket Doyma, New York, 151-157

Adams MR, Kaplan JR, Manuck SB, Koritnik DR, Parks JS, Wolfe MS, Clarkson TB (1990) Inhibition of coronary artery atherosclerosis by 17β-estradiol in ovariectomized monkeys. Lack of an effect of adding progesterone. Arteriosclerosis 10:1051-1057

Beldekas JC, Smith B, Geistenfeld LC (1981) Effects of 17-beta estradiol on the biosynthesis of collagen in cultured bovine aortic smooth muscle cells. Biochemistry 20:2161-2167

Bush TL (1990) The epidemiology of cardiovascular disease in postmenopausal women. Ann NY Acad Sci 592:263-271

Chang WC, Nakao J, Orimo H, Murota SI (1980) Stimulation of prostacyclin activity by estradiol in rat aorta smooth muscle cell in culture. Biochim Bioph Acta 619:107-118

Clarkson TB, Shively CA, Morgan TM, Koritnik DR, Adams MR, Kaplan JR (1990) Oral contraceptives and coronary artery atherosclerosis of cynomolgus monkeys. Obstet Gynecol 75:217-222

Engel HJ, Engel E, Lichtlen PR (1983) Coronary atherosclerosis and myocardial infarction in young women – role of oral contracepetives. Eur Heart J 4:1-8

Fischer GM (1972) In vivo effects of estradiol on collagen and elastin dynamics in rat aorta. Endocrinology 91:1227-1232

Fischer GM, Swain ML (1977) Effect of sex hormones on blood pressure and vascular connective tissue in castrated and noncastrated male rats. Am J Physiol 232:H617-H621

Fischer-Dzoga K, Wissler RW, Vesselinovitch D (1983) The effect of estradiol on the proliferation of rabbit aortic medial tissue culture cells induced by hyperlipemic serum. Exp Mol Pathol 39:355-363

Haarbo J, Leth-Espensen P, Stender S, Christiansen C (1991) Estrogen monotherapy and combined estrogen-progestogen replacement therapy attenuate aortic accumulation of cholesterol in ovariectomized cholesterol-fed rabbits. J Clin Invest 87:1274-1279

Hamm TE, Kaplan JR, Clarkson TB, Bullock BC (1983) Effects of gender and social behavior on the development of coronary artery atherosclerosis in cynomolgus monkeys. Atherosclerosis 221:48-57

Hough JL, Zilversmit DB (1986) Effect of 17-beta estradiol on aortic cholesterol content and metabolism in cholesterol-fed rabbits. Arteriosclerosis 6:57-63

Ingegno MD, Money SR, Thelmo W, Davidian M, Jaffe BM, Pertschuk, LP (1988) Progesterone receptors in the human heart and great vessels. Lab Invest 59:353-356

Johnson M, Ramey E, Ramwell PW (1977) Androgen-mediated sensitivity in platelet aggregation. Am J Physiol 232:H381-H385

Kaplan JR, Adams MR, Clarkson TB, Koritnik DR (1984) Psychosocial influences on female protection among cynomolgus macaques. Atherosclerosis 53:283-295

Lin AL, McGill HC, Shain SA (1982) Hormone receptors of the baboon cardiovascular system. Circ Res 50:610-616

Lin AL, Gonzalez R Jr, Carey KD, Shain SA (1986) Estradiol 17-beta affects estrogen receptor distribution and elevates progesterone receptor content in baboon aorta. Arteriosclerosis 6:495-504

McGill HC Jr, Stern MP (1979) Sex and atherosclerosis. Atherosclerosis Rev 4:157-242

McGill HC Jr, Axelrod LR, McMahan CA, et al. (1977) Estrogens and experimental atherosclerosis in the baboon (*Papio cynocephalus*). Circulation 56:657-662

Mishell DR Jr. (1988) Use of oral contraceptives in women of older reproductive age. Am J Obstet Gynecol 158:1652-1657

Pick R, Stamler J, Rodbard S, Katz LN (1952a) The inhibition of coronary atherosclerosis by estrogens in cholesterol-fed chicks. Circulation 6:276-280

Pick R, Stamler J, Rodbard S, Katz LN (1952b) Estrogen-induced regression of coronary atherosclerosis in cholesterol-fed chicks. Circulation 6:858-861

Prichard RW, Clarkson TB, Lofland HB (1966) Estrogen in pigeon atherosclerosis. Estradiol valerate effects at several dose levels on cholesterol-fed male White Carneau pigeons. Arch Pathol 82:15-17

Realini JP, Goldzieher JW (1985) Oral contraceptives and cardiovascular disease: A critique of the epidemiologic studies. Am J Obstet Gynecol 152:792-798

Rhee CY, Spaet TH, Gaynor E, et al. (1974) Suppression of surgically induced vascular intimal hypertrophy by estrogen. Circulation 49 (suppl III):III-92

Rhee CY, Drouet RO, Spaet YH, Geiger CH (1978) Growth inhibition of cultured vascular smooth muscle cells by estradiol. Fed Proc 37:474

Stamler J, Pick R, Katz LN (1954) Inhibition of cholesterol-induced coronary atherogenesis in the egg-producing hen. Circulation 10:251-254

Stampfer MJ, Willett WC, Colditz GA, Speizer FE, Hennekens CH (1990) Past use of oral contraceptives and cardiovascular disease: A meta-analysis in the context of the Nurses' Health Study. Am J Obstet Gynecol 163:285-291

Steinberg D, Parthasarathy S, Carew TE, Khoo JC, Witztum JL (1989) Beyond cholesterol. Modifications of low-density lipoprotein that increase its atherogenicity. N Engl J Med 320:915

Thorneycroft IH (1990) Oral contraceptives and myocardial infarction. Am J Obstet Gynecol 163:1393-1397

Thorogood M, Vessey MP (1990) An epidemiologic survey of cardiovascular disease in women taking oral contraceptives. Am J Obstet Gynecol 163:274-281

Wagner JD, Clarkson TB, Adams MR, Schwenke DC (1991) The effects of oral contraceptives on coronary artery LDL metabolism in female cynomolgus monkeys. Circulation 84 (Suppl II):II-602 (Abstract)

Wagner JD, Clarkson TB, St. Clair RW, Schwenke DC, Shively CA, Adams MR (1991) Estrogen and progesterone therapy reduces low density lipoprotein accumulation in the coronary arteries of surgically postmenopausal cynomolgus monkeys. J Clin Invest 88:1995-2002

Weigensberg BI, Lough H, More RH, Katz E, Pugash E, Peniston C (1984) Effects of estradiol on myointimal thickening from catheter injury and on organizing white mural nonocclusive thrombi. Atherosclerosis 52:253-265

Wolinsky H (1972) Effects of estrogen and progesterone treatment on the response of the aorta of male rats to hypertension. Circ Res 30:341-349

12 A Review of the Epidemiology of Postmenopausal Estrogens and the Risk of Coronary Heart Disease

Meir J. Stampfer

12.1 Introduction

Cardiovascular diseases, especially coronary heart disease, remain the leading cause of death in women. The rates are relatively low among premenopausal women, but rise sharply with age. Moreover, the ratio of rates between men and women grows smaller with increasing age (US Department of Health and Human Services 1988). This observation led to speculation that functioning ovaries in premenopausal women were protective. Although the risk of coronary heart disease (CHD) does not abruptly rise at the moment of natural menopause (Colditz et al. 1987; Stampfer et al. 1989), rates of heart disease increase substantially during the period of the climacteric. The increased risk of CHD among young women with bilateral oophorectomy (Stampfer et al. 1989) further supported the view that estrogens play an important role in reducing the risk of CHD in premenopausal women and that estrogen replacement therapy after menopause might decrease the risk.

This review summarizes the epidemiological evidence regarding the association between postmenopausal estrogen use and CHD. Substantial epidemiological evidence has accumulated from cross-sectional studies, hospital- and community-based case-control studies, prospective cohort studies, and a small clinical trial.

12.2 Hospital-Based Case-Control Studies

In this design, employed in six studies (Rosenberg et al. 1976, 1980; Jick et al. 1978a,b; Szklo et al. 1984; La Vecchia et al. 1987), estrogen use is ascertained among patients hospitalized for myocardial infarction (MI), and compared to that among other patients who serve as controls. This approach is often convenient and usually yields a high participation rate. However, there are some noteworthy limitations, including the possibility of recall bias. Another more difficult problem is proper selection of controls. It is essential to select controls from among patients diagnosed with diseases unrelated to estrogen use. This can be difficult because many diseases are related in some way to estrogen use. For example, in some studies, many of the controls were patients admitted for treatment of fracture. These studies were designed before it was widely appreciated that estrogens reduce osteoporosis and fracture. Such controls would be less likely to be estrogen users than comparably aged women in the population. Their inclusion in a study would tend to reduce the magnitude of the apparent inverse association between estrogens and risk of heart disease. Even exclusion of all diseases that are biologically related to estrogen use from the control pool may not completely solve this problem. For some patients, physicians may be reluctant to prescribe estrogens so as to avoid possible interactions with other medications or simply to avoid overburdening the patient with many different medications. Hence, the results could be biased even with a nonbiological behavioral link between disease status among the controls and likelihood of estrogen use.

Generally, the bias would be such that estrogen use in the controls would be reduced. Therefore, one would expect that hospital-based case-control studies might underestimate the reduction in risk of CHD due to estrogen. The relative risks observed in these studies range from 4.2 to 0.5. The results in most of the studies were generally null.

Jick et al. (1978b) reported one of the two case-control studies that observed an increased risk of coronary disease for apparently healthy estrogen users; the relative risk for estrogen use was 7.5. Limiting the findings to postmenopausal women yielded a relative risk of 4.2 (95% confidence interval (CI), 0.96–18.84). The study included only 14 cases among postmenopausal women; at least 13 were current cigarette smokers. In the larger study of which the results for postmenopausal women are a part, there was clearly a problem in enrolling subjects. Of 954 patients initially identified as eligible, only 95 were actually enrolled in the study; participation rates among controls were not given. This enrollment procedure may have introduced a bias. The small size of this study and the restriction to women under age 46 also render the findings difficult to interpret.

The other hospital-based case-control study was reported by La Vecchia et al. (1987). Cases were patients with a first nonfatal MI under age 55 drawn from 30 hospitals in Northern Italy. Controls were age-matched patients from the same hospitals being treated for conditions which were not cardiovascular, hormonal, or gynecologic in nature and were not related to cancer, cigarette smoking, or alcohol use. Forty percent of the controls had orthopedic disorders, many with fractures. Only 6% of controls and 8% of cases had ever used estrogens. The age-adjusted relative risk for current use was 2.95 (95% CI 0.80–10.80), and for past use, 0.77 (95% CI 0.16–3.60). The majority of cases (60%) and controls (58%) were premenopausal. No analysis was presented which included only postmenopausal women, and data are not provided in the paper to permit such a calculation. Hence, these results are difficult to interpret.

12.3 Population-Based Case-Control Studies

The population or community-based case-control studies (Talbott et al. 1977; Pfeffer et al. 1978; Ross et al. 1981; Bain et al. 1981; Adam et al. 1981; Beard et al. 1989; Thompson et al. 1989) share some of the methodological limitations of retrospective studies, including selection and enrollment of controls. However, this design does have the important advantage of avoiding the use of hospital controls. Hence, one would not expect a systematic underestimate of the effect of estrogens because the usage pattern among the controls would be expected to represent that of the population from which the MI cases were ascertained. The relative risks from these population-based case-control studies range from 0.3 to 0.9. All six studies of nonfatal MI observed an apparent protective effect of estrogens, but the reduction in risk was statistically significant in only one of them (Ross et al. 1981). A seventh case-control study (Thompson et al. 1989) reported on a combined endpoint of stroke and MI, with essentially null results.

In the largest community-based case-control study of MI, with 171 cases drawn from a California retirement community, Pfeffer et al. (1978) observed a relative risk of 0.7 (95% CI 0.3–1.4) among current users of estrogens. These investigators relied on pharmacy records to ascertain estrogen use. Although these records were thought to be nearly complete, in a later analysis (Ross et al. 1981) it was found that many women had estrogen use noted on their medical records despite having no record of a prescription in the retirement community pharmacy. This misclassification of estrogen use, if it were random with respect to case status, would tend to bias the results towards the null; this would reduce the power of the study to observe a benefit of estrogens if one were present, and underestimate the true effect. The mean duration of current use was less than 3 months for both cases and controls; this also would bias the findings towards an underestimate because many of the users would have had an insufficient duration of use to be of benefit.

In another case-control study in the same retirement community, Ross et al. (1981) used the medical records to assess use of estrogens by 133 residents who died of CHD. Apparently there was some overlap of cases with the previous study. For each case, one living and one dead control was matched by age, race and duration of residence in the community. Controls with a cause of death suspected to be associated with estrogen use were excluded. For ever use of estrogens, the relative risk was 0.43 (95% CI 0.24–0.75) compared with living controls and 0.57 (95% CI 0.33–0.99) compared with deceased controls. The apparent benefit was slightly more pronounced among women without notable coronary risk factors. They also found a suggestion of a greater benefit for a dose of 0.625 mg/day conjugated estrogens or less as compared with 1.25 mg/day or more. There was more apparent protection among nonsmokers or light smokers than among current smokers of one or more packs per day. There was essentially no change in relative risk estimates with multivariate adjustment, indicating a similar risk profile in users and nonusers in this population.

12.4 Cross-Sectional Studies

Table 1 summarizes the findings from three cross-sectional studies (Sullivan et al. 1988; Gruchow et al. 1988; McFarland et al. 1989). In each of these studies, the degree of coronary artery occlusion was assessed among users and nonusers of postmenopausal estrogens in women having coronary arteriography. This design has the advantage of avoiding recall bias and the problems of control selection and response bias that can appear in case-control studies. In this design, there is no loss to follow-up or misclassification of exposure status during follow-up that can occur in prospective cohort studies.

In all three studies, investigators compared the prevalence of estrogen use among women with severe occlusion (defined as 70% or more in two studies and as an average of 50% in the third study) with those with no stenosis. The results from all three studies were nearly identical; each observed a statistically significant decrease of about 60% for the risk of severe coronary disease among women using estrogens.

It is likely that this design would tend to overestimate the benefit of estrogen on CHD risk. Estrogen users, who have greater contact with the health care system, may be more likely to have angiography than nonusers with the same equivocal symptoms. Hence, the estrogen users in these studies may selectively be enriched with women without significant disease. Nonetheless, the magnitude of such a bias, if any, would be such that it could explain only a small fraction of the appar-

Table 1. Age- and multiple risk factor-adjusted relative risks (RR) of cardio-vascular diseases among current and past postmenopausal hormone users compared with those who never used postmenopausal hormones.

Use category	Person-years		Major coronary disease		Fatal cardiovascular disease	
			Cases	RR (95% CI)	Cases	RR (95% CI)
Never	179	194	250	1.0 (referent)	129	1.0 (referent)
Current	73	532				
Age-adjusted			45	0.51 (0.37-0.70)	21	0.48 (0.31-0.74)
Age- and risk factor-adjusted				0.56 (0.40-0.80)		0.61 (0.37-1.00)
Past	85	128				
Age-adjusted			110	0.91 (0.73-1.14)	55	0.84 (0.61-1.15)
Age- and risk factor-adjusted				0.83 (0.65-1.05)		0.79 (0.56-1.10)

Risk factors included in the multivariate models are age, cigarette smoking, hypertension, diabetes, high serum cholesterol, parental history of MI below age 60, Quetelet's index, past oral contraceptive use, and time period

ent benefit of estrogen observed in these studies. In their study, Gruchow et al. (1988) specifically addressed this issue and found that estrogen users and nonusers had an identical pattern of symptoms, suggesting the absence of any bias.

In Gruchow's study, controlling for total cholesterol and triglyceride levels in the regression model had no material effect on the magnitude or statistical significance of the inverse association between estrogen use and coronary occlusion. However, when high-density lipoprotein (HDL) cholesterol was added to the model, it substantially reduced that association. This effect is consistent with the view that elevations in HDL (and a decrease in LDL) are the most likely mechanisms of action for the apparent benefit of estrogen. In most analyses, it is inappropriate to adjust for these variables since they are in the causal pathway for estrogens. When one controls for HDL, it is equivalent to asking what the effect of estrogen is on coronary risk above and beyond the effect on HDL levels.

12.5 Prospective Studies

Results from 14 prospective studies (Potocki 1971; Burch et al. 1974; McMahon 1978; Hammond et al. 1979; Nachtigall et al. 1979; Lafferty and Helmuth 1985; Stampfer et al. 1985; Wilson et al. 1985; Eaker and Castelli 1987; Bush et al. 1983, 1987; Petitti et al. 1987; Hunt et al. 1987; Criqui et al. 1988; Henderson et al. 1988; Croft and Hannaford 1989) have been published. One is a small clinical trial (Nachtigall et al. 1979) and the rest are observational studies. In principle, prospective studies have important advantages over case-control studies in avoiding recall bias and the difficulties of control selection and participation. Apart from confounding, the chief bias is likely to result from differential follow-up (i.e., an MI would be missed among estrogen users with a different‚probability than among nonusers). This did not appear to be a serious problem in the studies reviewed here. Another potential problem with prospective studies is that often estrogen use is ascertained at baseline, and this exposure information is not updated during subsequent follow-up for CHD. If estrogen use was changing during the follow-up, then the resulting misclassification would cause an underestimate of the effect of estrogen. This problem may be particularly acute because the benefits of estrogen are most pronounced among current or recent users. All of the prospective studies have observed a protective effect of estrogens for CHD risk, though the results from the Framingham Study are equivocal (Wilson et al. 1985; Eaker and Castelli 1987).

One may distinguish two types of prospective studies by the presence or absence of an internal comparison group. Most of the studies followed up women with and without estrogen exposure, and thus had an internal control group. Such a design is preferable because the exposed and unexposed individuals are generally comparable. In three of the prospective studies (Burch et al. 1974; Hunt et al. 1987; McMahon 1978), the entire cohort was taking estrogens. The mortality experience is then compared with national statistics to derive a relative risk. In most instances, patients given estrogen will be healthier than the general population, in part by virtue of their connection with the medical care system. Although these studies can have estrogen exposure misclassification that would attenuate the benefit, the bias due to a comparison with general population statistics is probably more important, so that these studies probably overstate the benefit of estrogen. The relative risk in each of these studies was approximately 0.3.

The only randomized trial of estrogens was reported by Nachtigall et al. (1979) in 84 matched pairs of chronic disease hospital patients. In each pair, one patient was given placebo and the other was given 2.5 mg/day conjugated estrogen with 10 mg/day medroxyprogesterone added for 7 days each month. After 10 years of follow-up, there were only four cases of MI, one in the treatment group and three in the placebo group, for a relative risk of 0.33 (95% CI 0.04–2.82). For total mortality, the relative risk was 0.43 (95% CI 0.12–1.54). Although the design was sound, the small size of the study is a serious limitation.

Another small but long-term prospective study was reported by Lafferty and Helmuth (1985), who followed up 61 estrogen users and 63 nonusers aged 45–60 years for a mean of 8.6 years. At baseline, all women were considered eligible for and were offered estrogen therapy, but 63 declined; they formed the comparison group. Of the 74 estrogen users, 61 used estrogens (0.6 mg/day conjugated estrogens for 3 weeks per month, with no progestins) for a minimum of 3 years and constituted the estrogen-treated group. The remaining 13 discontinued estrogen after a short time; none had any complications. Of the seven MIs that were diagnosed during follow-up, six were in the control group and only one was in the estrogen group, for a relative risk of 0.17 (95% CI 0.03–1.06). The incidence of angina was the same in both groups, with two cases each. In addition, there were five cases of new ECG abnormalities in the control group as compared with two in the estrogen group. Thus, the relative risk for any abnormal ECG change was 0.28 (95% CI 0.09–0.87). The risk factor distribution was quite similar in both groups, but the estrogen users tended to be somewhat leaner.

The Nurses' Health Study (Stampfer et al. 1985) is the largest prospective cohort study to address this issue. The study was established in 1976 when 121 700 married female registered nurses aged 30–55 years completed a mailed questionnaire that included items about health status, medical history, and a variety of life-style practices, including hormone use and a variety of coronary risk factors. Information on risk factors and hormone use was updated by means of follow-up questionnaires sent every 2 years. A total of 32 317 postmenopausal women without prior CHD were followed up for an average of 3 years for a total follow-up of 105 786 person-years. Current users of estrogens had a relative risk of 0.3 (95% CI 0.2–0.6). Among past users, there was a relative risk of 0.7, but this did not attain statistical significance, with 95% CI of 0.4–1.2. There was no material effect of duration or dose, and the findings were essentially unchanged after adjustment for a variety of coronary risk factors.

A recent update from the Nurses' Health Study (Stampfer et al. 1991b) reported on endpoints of nonfatal MI and fatal CHD with 10 years of follow-up. We accrued 337 854 person-years among 48 470 postmenopausal women during this 10-year period. Follow-up for non-fatal outcomes was 88.4% complete, and for mortality, more than 98% complete.

For each participant, information on exposure variables was up-dated according to subsequent questionnaire responses; follow-up ended with a diagnosis of cardiovascular disease or death. Information on exposures and other possible risk factors is derived from self-report, but we believe it to be reliable. Substudies have validated self-reports by review of medical records and direct measurement for several conditions (Colditz et al. 1986), and the subjects are all registered nurses with a demonstrated interest in medical research. Current, past and never users had basically similar patterns of distribution of potential cardiovascular disease risk factors.

During the 10-year follow-up period, among the postmenopausal women free from prior cardiovascular disease we documented 293 nonfatal MIs and 112 confirmed coronary deaths. The age-adjusted risk for major coronary disease among current users was about half that of never users, with a relative risk of 0.51 (95% CI 0.37–0.70; $p < 0.0001$) (Table 1). Among past users, the age-adjusted relative risk was 0.91 (95% CI 0.73–1.14; $p = 0.42$).

We found no notable trends among past users with regard to duration of use or time since last use, and no evidence suggesting that the degree of protection associated with current estrogen use was related to duration of use. The most strongly supported mechanism for this effect is the obvious favorable impact of estrogens on lipids: estrogens raise HDL cholesterol and lower LDL-cholesterol. Although estrogen-induced changes in lipid metabolism are adequate to explain a large reduction in risk of coronary disease (Bush et al. 1986), other possible mechanisms have been proposed (Lobo 1990). We found less benefit among women taking more than 1.25 mg daily. Such high doses were common in the Framingham cohort, which may partly explain their discrepant results (see below).

Among women who had a natural menopause, the age-adjusted relative risk of major coronary disease among current users was 0.62 (95% CI 0.39–0.97), similar but somewhat less extreme than that among women with bilateral oophorectomy, at 0.40 (95% CI 0.22–0.73).

To assess the effect of estrogen use among low risk women, we defined a subgroup of women who had no diagnosis of hypertension, diabetes, or high serum cholesterol, were not current smokers, and had a Quetelet's index below 32 kg/m^2. For this group, the age-adjusted relative risk for major coronary disease among current users was 0.53 (95% CI 0.31–0.91). This suggests that lower risk women enjoy the same relative benefit as women in general. However, because coronary disease rates are lower among the low risk women, the same relative decrease corresponds to a smaller reduction in the number of events.

We adjusted for the effects of several potential risk factors simultaneously by using proportional hazards models to estimate the relative risks of current and past use of estrogens, controlling for age, follow-up interval, and various self-reported characteristics. Because current estrogen users were somewhat healthier, this adjustment slightly diminished the apparent benefit. The results were similar to those adjusted for age alone; for major coronary disease, the relative risk among current users was 0.56 (95% CI 0.40–0.80).

To evaluate whether increased medical care of women using postmenopausal estrogens might be responsible for the benefit, we limited the analysis to women who reported a physician visit in 1978 (65% of the cohort). The results were similar to the larger population: the age-adjusted relative risk for major CHD was 0.45 (95% CI 0.31–0.66) for current use, and 0.79 (95% CI 0.60–1.05) for past use.

The Framingham Heart Study (Wilson et al. 1985), unlike all the other cohort studies, reported an increase in risk of cardiovascular disease among ever users of estrogen. If estrogen was included on the medication form completed during the biennial examinations during an 8-year period (examinations 8–12), a participant was classified as a user of estrogen. Follow-up began at the end of that 8-year interval (i.e., at examination 12) for 1234 postmenopausal women 50 years of age or older and extended for an additional 8 years (i.e., examinations

13–16). Among these women, 302 had used estrogens at some time. After controlling for age, HDL-cholesterol, hypertension, obesity, total cholesterol, smoking, and alcohol use, the relative risk for all cardiovascular disease among ever users of estrogen was 1.8 compared with never users. The category of total cardiovascular disease included nearly all possible manifestations: CHD, angina pectoris, intermittent claudication, transient ischemic attack, MI, congestive heart failure and coronary and sudden death. In spite of this apparent increase in risk, and in spite of the fact that cardiovascular disease is the leading cause of death in women of that age, there was no effect on total mortality, with a relative risk of 1.0. When only MI was considered ($n = 51$ cases), the apparent increase in risk (RR = 1.87) was not statistically significant. This apparent increase in risk was concentrated among smokers, in whom a significant effect was observed both for total cardiovascular disease and for MI.

A second analysis of the Framingham data (Eaker and Castelli 1987) demonstrated that the results were quite sensitive to the choice of the baseline examination. Eaker et al. state that "after careful analysis of the data, it was evident that the relationships observed between estrogen use or nonuse and cardiovascular disease were present only for examination 12" (Eaker and Castelli 1987). The second analysis (Eaker and Castelli 1987) was limited to CHD without angina and considered two time periods instead of just one (i.e., using examinations 11 and 12 as the baselines for assessing estrogen use for the subsequent 10-year follow-up). Taking the average of the findings using the two baselines, there was a nonsignificant protective effect among women aged 50 to 59 years, with a relative risk of 0.38 (95% CI 0.06–2.29). Among older women, there was a nonsignificant adverse effect, with a relative risk of 1.82 (95% CI 0.48–6.89). In both Framingham analyses, the results were adjusted for HDL cholesterol. As discussed earlier, this is generally inappropriate.

Findings from the Lipid Research Clinics were reported by Bush et al. (1987) based on follow-up of 2270 women aged 40–69 years at baseline when estrogen use was ascertained. After 8 years of follow-up (without further updating of estrogen use), the age-adjusted relative risk of cardiovascular death among current estrogen users compared with nonusers was 0.34 (95% CI 0.12–0.81). Controlling for other coronary risk factors which may have confounded the association, including age, blood pressure, smoking, and prior cardiovascular disease, had little impact on this estimate, yielding a relative risk of 0.37 (95% CI 0.16–0.88), demonstrating that estrogen users and nonusers in this cohort had similar distributions of coronary risk factors, except obesity (estrogen users were leaner) and HDL (users had higher levels). This issue was examined in detail (Bush et al. 1983, 1987); users and non-users had a similar pattern of personal and family history of cardiovas-cular disease, risk factors, and use of cardiovascular medications.

The Leisure World Study was the largest in terms of number of out-comes (Henderson et al. 1988). In this study, 8841 women aged 40-101 years living in a retirement community completed a health survey questionnaire in 1981. In the ensuing 5 years (40 919 person-years), 1019 deaths (149 due to MI) occurred. The relative risk for ever users of estrogen as compared with never users for all-cause mortality was 0.8 (95% CI 0.70–0.91). The majority of this reduction in the total death rate was due to a lower level of the rate of fatal MI; the relative risk for ever users of estrogens was 0.59 (95% CI 0.42–0.82). Past or current estrogen use was distinguished on the baseline questionnaire. For past users the relative risk was 0.62, and for current users, 0.47. There was no further update of information on estrogen use after the baseline questionnaire. Control for a wide variety of potential con-founding factors, including prior coronary disease, hypertension, smoking, obesity, and exercise, had little or no impact on the relative risk estimates. Estrogen had a similar benefit within categories of these risk factors except for current smokers, in whom no protection was ob-served (but this was based on only 17 cases), and older age at last men-strual period (based on 14 cases). There was no material difference in protection according to hysterectomy status, and there was no apparent dose or duration effect. The women in this study were considerably older, on average, than those in most other studies, with a median age of 73 years.

The results from all these studies were combined in a meta-analysis (Stampfer et al. 1991a). Of the 29 studies evaluated, two were null (relative risks between 0.9 and 1.1), and four showed an adverse trend. In none of the latter was the adverse effect statistically significant. Among the 23 studies that found a reduced risk of CHD among es-trogen users, the results in 11 were statistically significant. The relative risks for all studies ranged from 0.17 to 4.2.

The first meta-analysis included all studies, whenever possible using estimates for ever use. This yielded a summary estimated relative risk of 0.56. The summary relative risks within types of study design are statistically incompatible. In contrast to the other designs, the hospital-based case-control studies tended to show a nonsignificant trend toward an adverse effect of estrogens, with a summary relative risk of 1.33 (95% CI 0.93–1.91). All other designs show statistically significant reductions in risk. A summary estimate of all studies except the hospital-based case-control studies yielded a relative risk of 0.52. The most plausible estimates are provided by the cohort studies with internal controls, with a relative risk of 0.58 (95% CI 0.48–0.70).

12.6 Factors Which May Modify the Effect of Estrogens on CHD Risk

In addition to assessing the association between ever use of estrogens and risk of CHD, several studies have also explored factors that could modify this association, including recency of use, duration, type of hormone preparation, and dose, as well as particular subgroups of women in whom the degree of benefit may be altered, such as by age, type of menopause, and cigarette smoking habits.

Current users of estrogens appeared to enjoy greater protection than past or ever users. The studies by Rosenberg et al. (1976, 1980), Pfeffer et al. (1978), and Bain et al. (1981) found a lower relative risk for current users. Only the study by Adam et al. (1981) found a (nonsignificantly) higher risk, but this was based on only two cases in the current use category. Only two of the prospective studies directly compared these two groups. Henderson et al. (1988) observed a relative risk of 0.47 for current use and 0.62 for past use. Stampfer et al. (1985) reported a relative risk of 0.30 for current use and 0.59 for past use. A summary of these two yielded a relative risk of 0.37 (95% CI 0.21–0.65) for current use and 0.61 (95% CI 0.45–0.84) for past use. In all three cross-sectional studies, the use was defined as current. In many of the cohort studies, current use was defined at baseline and not updated, leading to misclassification of the exposure variable, which attenuated the relative risk. The difference in effect of current or recent use and past use may partly explain the greater apparent protection in the cross-sectional studies.

Few studies have examined the effects of duration of use of estrogens on risk of CHD. Both Henderson et al. (1988) and Stampfer et al. (1985, 1991b) mentioned that they observed no effect of duration.

The type of hormone preparation has generally not been studied specifically. Most investigations were conducted in the United States, where oral conjugated estrogens (specifically Premarin) were by far the most common form of estrogen used. Only in the two British studies was Premarin use not predominant: the population-based study by Thompson et al. (1989), with null findings, and the uncontrolled cohort study by Hunt et al. (1987), in which a benefit of estrogen was observed.

Few reports have provided data on the effects of different doses. Ross et al. (1981) found a nonsignificant trend for greater protection from doses of 0.625 mg/day of conjugated estrogens than from 1.25 mg/day or more. However, Henderson et al. (1988), in a later prospective study in the same population, found no effect of dose, in agreement with Stampfer et al. (1985) in the Nurses' Health Study.

Apart from the particulars of the exposure to estrogens, there is also interest in whether the benefits may differ in different subgroups of women. Age has been suggested as a possibly important modifier of the effect, especially since a trend towards benefit was observed in the Framingham study for younger women, while a nonsignificant adverse effect was seen in those over age 60. Stampfer et al. (1985) and Bush et al. (1983) observed a benefit at all ages in their studies. Sullivan et al. (1988) found slightly greater protection among younger women, while Gruchow et al. (1988) found the opposite; in both studies, all age groups experienced an apparent benefit. The study by Henderson et al. (1988) is especially important in this regard; they observed substantial benefit in their population with a median age of 73 years.

The effect of type of menopause was investigated in several studies. Gruchow et al. (1988) and Henderson et al. (1988) found no differences. Bain et al. (1981) found a protective effect only among those with bilateral oophorectomy in a fairly young population (under age 55); in all the other studies, a benefit was observed regardless of type of menopause, but the magnitude of protection was greater among those with a surgical menopause (Szklo et al. 1984; McFarland et al. 1989; Stampfer et al. 1985; Bush et al. 1983).

Several studies have observed more protection from estrogens among nonsmokers or light smokers (Ross et al. 1981; Sullivan et al. 1988; Henderson et al. 1988). Wilson et al. (1985) observed no effect among nonsmokers and an adverse effect of estrogens among smokers. Criqui et al. (1988) observed the opposite, with a benefit only among current smokers, and an adverse effect among past smokers.

12.7 Association of Estrogens with Lower Risk of CHD: Cause and Effect or Selection?

The finding that estrogen users are at lower risk from coronary disease does not necessarily imply cause and effect. Patients and their physicians decide upon estrogen therapy, and often the health status of the patient will have an important influence.

Some have argued that estrogen use is merely a marker rather than a cause of good health. Most of the studies have provided some information bearing on this critical point. One way to judge the evidence for this position is to examine results of studies in which all the women were judged eligible by their physicians to receive estrogens. Only two small studies meet that criterion (Lafferty and Helmuth 1985; Stampfer et al. 1985); the summary relative risk from those two was 0.22 (95% CI 0.06–0.88). These findings do not support the hypothesis that selection of healthy women for estrogen use can explain the lower rate of CHD among estrogen users.

Another approach is to examine the risk profile of estrogen users and nonusers to determine whether there is a consistent pattern of higher risk among the nonusers, and to assess whether the differences, if any, are sufficient to explain the large decrease in risk among estrogen users. In the Nurses' Health Study, the distribution of established coronary risk factors was quite similar among current and never users of estrogens (Stampfer et al. 1985). Similar findings were observed in the Lipid Research Clinics Follow-up Study (Bush et al. 1987); Table 2 summarizes the results from those two studies which examined this issue in detail. In both studies, multivariate control for risk factors had almost no effect on the relative risk, implying an equivalent risk status for users and nonusers. As noted earlier, in the Nurses' Health Study, a similar degree of benefit was observed when the

Table 2. Risk factor profile of estrogen users and nonusers

Stampfer et al. 1985 Prevalence (%) of coronary risk factors by estrogen use			Bush et al. 1987 Mean level or prevalence of risk factor by estrogen use		
Variable	Never	Current	Characteristic	Nonuser	User
Maternal MI	11	11	Age (years)	53	54
Paternal MI	23	25	Systolic BP	128	129
Smoking	38	35	Diastolic BP	80	80
Hypertension[a]	18	18	Body mass index (kg/m^2)	26	25
High cholesterol[a]	5	6	Cholesterol (mg/dl)	235	235
Diabetes[a]	3	2	Smoking (%)	31	33
Body mass index $> 24.6 \, kg/m^2$	42	32	Regular exercise	10	12
			Alcohol use (%)	79	82

[a] By self-report

analysis was limited to women with a recent visit to a physician or when only women at low risk for CHD were assessed.

An indirect approach to this issue is to examine the direction and magnitude of change in the relative risk in moving from age-adjusted to age- and risk factor-adjusted estimates. No change implies no difference in the risk factor profiles between estrogen users and nonusers. If the relative risk decreases, this implies that users were at higher baseline risk from other coronary risk factors, whereas if it increases, it implies a lower coronary risk profile among the users. All three findings have been observed. Besides the studies of Stampfer et al. (1985) and Bush et al. (1987) in which multivariate analysis had little effect on the relative risk, similarly no such effect was observed by McFarland et al. (1989), Ross et al. (1981), Henderson et al. (1988) or (Croft and Hannaford (1989). In the studies by Sullivan et al. (1988), Bain et al. (1981), Rosenberg et al. (1976), Thompson et al. (1989) and Criqui et al. (1988), the relative risk estimates increased slightly after multivariate analysis. In general, the change was modest; the largest difference was in the hospital case-control study by Rosenberg et al. (1976), where the relative risk went from 0.71 to 0.97. On the other

Table 3. Risk factor profile in estrogen users compared to nonusers

Somewhat lower	Slightly lower	The same	Slightly higher	Somewhat higher
Hammond	Sullivan	Gruchow	Szklo	Rosenberg (1980)
Criqui	Lafferty	McFarland	Bain	Petitti
Rosenberg (1976)	Thompson	Ross		
Wilson		Adam		
		Stampfer		
		Bush		
		Henderson		
		Croft		
		Nachtigall		

hand, Petitti et al. (1987) found that multivariate control revealed an even stronger protective effect, which could occur only if estrogen users had a somewhat higher underlying risk; the estimate changed from 0.9 to 0.6. Szklo et al. (1984) and Rosenberg et al. (1980) also found a decrease in the relative risk following multivariate analysis. Thus, the findings are inconsistent. In some populations the risk of CHD for estrogen users and nonusers are essentially the same, and in others it varies in either direction (Table 3). There are thus substantial data to suggest that no more than a small portion of the benefit of estrogen can be explained by selection of healthier women for estrogen use.

A plausible biological mechanism for the protective effect of estrogen is its impact on the lipid profile. Among postmenopausal women, estrogens lower the levels of LDL-cholesterol and raise the concentration of HDL-cholesterol (Bush et al. 1986). Lower levels of LDL and elevated levels of HDL are both associated with reduced risk of heart disease. Estrogens can have a marked impact on both lipid fractions. Bush and Miller (1986) reviewed a substantial body of experimental work and found that on average, 0.625 mg/day of conjugated estrogens led to a 10% increase in HDL and a 4% decrease in LDL. Other forms of oral estrogen had generally similar effects. A 1 mg/dl increase in HDL is associated with approximately a 3–5% decrease in risk of coronary disease, and a 1 mg/dl decrease in LDL is associated with about a 2% decline in risk; hence, the changes induced by estrogen could lead to a relatively large decrease in risk (Gordon et al. 1989).

The effects of estrogen on the lipid profile begin within weeks of initiating therapy and do not persist after therapy is terminated. This may explain the consistent finding of a stronger protective effect for current use than for ever or past use. Most of the prospective studies did not reclassify the subjects' estrogen use during follow-up. If subjects ceased using estrogens during the follow-up (as many would be expected to do), this would lead to misclassification and consequently to an underestimate of the magnitude of protection. Criqui et al. (1988) discussed this point clearly in the analysis of their findings.

It is likely that other mechanisms of estrogen are active. Estrogen receptors are found throughout the cardiovascular system, and estrogen improves blood flow. In studies in monkeys, Adams et al. (1990) observed a marked decrease in atherosclerosis in oophorectomized monkeys given estrogens; only part of the effect was due to lipid changes. There was a marked reduction in LDL uptake in vessel walls (Wagner et al. 1991). Still other mechanisms involving vascular reactivity and prostaglandin changes have been proposed.

Progestin use was quite uncommon during the period that most of the epidemiological studies were conducted. Hence, most of the data relate directly to use of estrogens alone. Progestins are often prescribed along with estrogens to reduce or eliminate the excess risk of endometrial cancer due to unopposed estrogen. Unfortunately, progestins tend to have an effect on lipids opposite to that of estrogen: progestins tend to raise LDL and lower HDL. In women without a uterus, this consideration would be irrelevant.

The preponderance of evidence from the epidemiologic studies strongly supports the view that postmenopausal estrogen therapy can substantially reduce the risk for CHD. Widespread use of estrogen is likely to have a major beneficial impact in reducing CHD in women.

References

Adam S, Williams V, Vessey MP (1981) Cardiovascular disease and hormone replacement treatment: a pilot case-control study. Br Med J 282:1277-1278

Adams MR, Kaplan JR, Manuck SB, Koritnik DR, Parks JS, Wolfe MS, Clarkson TB (1990) Inhibition of coronary artery atherosclerosis by 17-beta estradiol in ovariectomized monkeys. Lack of an effect of added progesterone. Arteriosclerosis 10:1051-1057

Bain C, Willett WC, Hennekens CH, Rosner B, Belanger C, Speizer FE (1981) Use of postmenopausal hormones and risk of myocardial infarction. Circulation 64:42-46

Beard CM, Kottke TE, Annegers JF, Ballard DJ (1989) The Rochester Coronary Heart Disease Project: impact of cigarette smoking, hypertension, diabetes, and steroidal estrogen use on coronary heart disease among 40-59 year old women, 1960-82. Mayo Clinic Proc (in press)

Burch JC, Byrd Jr BF, Vaughn WK (1974) The effects of long-term estrogen on hysterectomized women. Am J Obstet Gynecol 188:778-782

Bush TL, Miller VT (1986) Effects of pharmacologic agents used during menopause. Impact on lipids and lipoproteins. In: Mishell D (ed) Menopause: physiology and pharmacology. Year Book Medical Publishers, Chicago, pp 187-208

Bush TL, Cowan LD, Barrett-Connor E, Criqui M, Karon JM, Wallace RB, Tyroler HA, Rifkind BM (1983) Estrogen use and all-cause mortality: preliminary results from the Lipid Research Clinics Program Follow-up Study. JAMA 249:903-906

Bush TL, Barrett-Connor E, Cowan LD, Criqui MH, Wallace RB, Suchindran CM, Tyroler HA, Rifkind BM (1987) Cardiovascular mortality and non-contraceptive use of estrogen in women: results from the Lipid Research Clinics Program Follow-up Study. Circulation 75:1102-1109

Colditz GA, Martin P, Stampfer MJ, Willett WC, Sampson L, Rosner B, Hennekens CH, Speizer FE (1986) Validation of questionnaire on risks factors and disease outcomes in a prospective cohort study in women. Am J Epidemiol 123:894-900

Colditz GA, Willett WC, Stampfer MJ, Rosner B, Speizer FE, Hennekens CH (1987) Menopause and the risk of coronary heart disease in women. N Engl J Med 316:1105-1110

Criqui MH, Suarez L, Barrett-Connor E, McPhillips J, Wingard DL, Garland C (1988) Postmenopausal estrogen use and mortality. Am J Epidemiol 128:606-614

Croft P, Hannaford PC (1989) Risk factors for acute myocardial infarction in women: evidence from the Royal College of General Practitioners' oral contraceptive study. Br Med J 298:165-168

Eaker ED, Castelli WP (1987) Coronary heart disease and its risk factors among women in the Framingham Study. In: Eaker E, Packard B, Wenger

NK, Clarkson TB, Tyroler HA (eds) Coronary heart disease in women. Haymarket Doyma Inc., New York, pp 122-132

Gordon DJ, Probstfield JL, Garrison RJ, Neaton JD, Castelli WP, Knoke JD, Jacobs Jr DR, Bangdiwala S, Tyroler HA (1989) High-density lipoprotein cholesterol and cardiovascular disease. Four prospective American studies. Circulation 79:8-15

Gruchow HW, Anderson AJ, Barboriak JJ, Sobocinski KA (1988) Postmenopausal use of estrogen and occlusion of coronary arteries. Am Heart J 115:954-963

Hammond CB, Jelovsek FR, Lee LK, Creasman WT, Parker RT (1979) Effects of long-term estrogen replacement therapy. I: Metabolic effects. Am J Obstet Gynecol 133:525-536

Henderson BE, Paganini-Hill A, Ross RK (1988) Estrogen replacement therapy and protection from acute myocardial infarction. Am J Obstet Gynecol 159:312-317

Hunt K, Vessey M, McPherson K, Coleman M (1987) Long-term surveillance of mortality and cancer incidence in women receiving hormone replacement therapy. Br J Obstet Gynecol 94:620-635

Jick H, Dinan B, Herman R, Rothman KJ (1978) Myocardial infarction and other vascular diseases in young women: role of estrogens and other factors. JAMA 240:2548-2552

Jick H, Dinan B, Rothman KJ (1978) Noncontraceptive estrogens and nonfatal myocardial infarction. JAMA 239:1407-1408

Lafferty FW, Helmuth DO (1985) Postmenopausal estrogen replacement: the prevention of osteoporosis and systemic effects. Maturitas 7:147-159

La Vecchia C, Franceschi S, Decarli A, Pampallona S, Tognoni G (1987) Risk factors for myocardial infarction in young women. Am J Epidemiol 125:832-843

Lobo RA (1990) Estrogen and cardiovascular disease. Ann NY Acad Sci 592:286-294

McFarland KF, Boniface ME, Hornung CA, Earnhardt W, Humphries JO (1989) Risk factors and noncontraceptive estrogen use in women with and without coronary disease. Am Heart J 117:1209-1214

McMahon B (1978). Cardiovascular disease and noncontraceptive oestrogen therapy. In: Oliver MF (ed) Coronary heart disease in young women. Churchill Livingstone, New York, pp 197-207

Nachtigall LE, Nachtigall RH, Nachtigall RD, Beckman EM (1979) Estrogen replacement therapy II: a prospective study in the relationship to carcinoma and cardiovascular and metabolic problems. Obstet Gynecol 54:74-79

Petitti DB, Perlman JA, Sidney S (1987) Noncontraceptive estrogens and mortality: long-term follow-up of women in the Walnut Creek Study. Obstet Gynecol 70:289-293

Pfeffer RI, Whipple GH, Kurosaki TT, Chapman JM (1978) Coronary risk and estrogen use in postmenopausal women. Am J Epidemiol 107:479-487

Potocki J (1971) Wplyw leczenia estrogenami na niewydolnose wiencowa u kobiet po menopauzie. Pol Tyg Lek 26:1812-1815

Rosenberg L, Armstrong B, Jick H (1976) Myocardial infarction and estrogen therapy in postmenopausal women. N Engl J Med 294:1256-1259

Rosenberg L, Stone D, Shapiro S, Kaufman P, Stolley PD, Miettinen OS (1980) Noncontraceptive estrogens and myocardial infarction in young women. JAMA 244:339-342

Ross RK, Paganini-Hill A, Mack TM, Arthur M, Henderson BE (1981) Menopausal oestrogen therapy and protection from death from ischaemic heart disease. Lancet 1:858-860

Stampfer MJ, Colditz GA (1991) Estrogen replacement therapy and coronary heart disease: a quantitative assessment of the epidemiologic evidence. Prev Med 20:47-63

Stampfer MJ, Willett WC, Colditz GA, Rosner B, Speizer FE, Hennekens CH (1985) A prospective study of postmenopausal estrogen therapy and coronary heart disease. N Engl J Med 313:1044-1049

Stampfer MJ, Colditz GA, Willett WC (1989) Menopause and heart disease: a review. Ann NY Acad Sci (in press)

Stampfer MJ, Colditz GA, Willett WC, Manson JE, Rosner B, Speizer FE, Hennekens CH (1991) Postmenopausal estrogen therapy and cardiovascular disease: ten-year follow-up from the Nurses' Health Study. N Engl J Med 325:756-762

Sullivan JM, Zwagg RV, Lemp GF, Hughes JP, Maddock V, Kroetz FW, Ramanathan KB, Mirvis DM (1988) Postmenopausal estrogen use and coronary atherosclerosis. Ann Int Med 108:358-363

Szklo M, Tonascia J, Gordis L, Bloom I (1984) Estrogen use and myocardial infarction risk: a case-control study. Prev Med 13:510-516

Talbott E, Kuller LH, Detre K, Perper J (1977) Biologic and psychosocial risk factors of sudden death from coronary disease in white women. Am J Cardiol 39:858-864

Thompson SG, Meade TW, Greenberg G (1989) The use of hormonal replacement therapy and the risk of stroke and myocardial infarction in women. J Epidemiol Comm Health 43:173-178

US Department of Health and Human Services, Public Health Service, Centers for Disease Control, National Center for Health Statistics (1988) Vital statistics of the United States 1986. Vol II: Mortality, part A. Hyattsville, Maryland

Wagner JD, Clarkson TB, St. Clair RW, Schwenke DC, Shively CA, Adams MR (1991) Estrogen and progesterone replacement therapy reduces low density lipoprotein accumulation in the coronary artery of surgically postmenopausal cynomolgus monkeys. J Clin Invest 88:1995-2002

Wilson PW, Garrison RJ, Castelli WP (1985) Postmenopausal estrogen use, cigarette smoking, and cardiovascular morbidity in women over 50: the Framingham Study. N Engl J Med 313:1038-1043

Subject Index